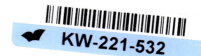

Trans Fats
Alternatives

Editors

Dharma R. Kodali
Global Agritech Inc.
Minneapolis, Minnesota

Gary R. List
USDA, NCAUR
Peoria, Illinois

AOCS
PRESS

Champaign, Illinois

AOCS Mission Statement
To be the global forum for professionals interested in lipids and related materials through the exchange of ideas, information, science, and technology.

Library of Congress Cataloging-in-Publication Data

Trans fats alternatives / edited by Dharma R. Kodali, Gary R. List
    p. cm.
  Includes bibliographical references and index.
  ISBN 1-893997-52-9 (alk. paper)
  1. Food--Fat content. 2. Trans fatty acids. I. Kodali, Dharma R., 1951- II. List, Gary R.

TX553.L5T73 2005
613.2'84--dc22

2005007957

CIP

Printed in the United States of America.
08 07 06 5 4 3 2

Preface

The date January 1, 2006, is significant to all of us in the fats and oils industry. On that date, the Food and Drug Administration (FDA) will require the mandatory declaration of the amount of *trans* fat present in foods. The regulations do not require food product manufacturers to reformulate their products to reduce/eliminate *trans* fats, but it requires declaring the amount of *trans* fat in grams per serving on the "Nutrition Facts" label. Since the FDA *trans* fats ruling two years ago, extensive media coverage around the country has made the public aware of *trans* fats and their influence on heart disease. The negative perception associated with *trans* fats has strongly influenced the food product manufacturers to eliminate or reduce the *trans* fats in their products. Scientists around the world are working to create solutions or alternatives to the *trans* fat dilemma. In an effort to address this problem at this critical juncture, we have gathered the best in the fats and oils business to create this compendium to educate public and pundits of fats and oils alike to deal with the new *trans* fat labeling requirements.

This book is principally for everyone who is interested to know more about *trans* fats, food product manufacturers who would like to provide the *trans* fat solutions and to the researchers who would like to create innovative solutions. Part of the inspiration and the subject matter for this book comes from a one day symposium on "*trans* FATS Food for Thought" that took place in Chicago a year ago. Fats and oils processors, food product manufacturers, and researchers from industry, academia and government attended this symposium. We hope this book will draw attention from a broad non-technical and technical audience.

The contents of this book can be divided into three parts. Chapters 1 to 3 covers the background and the fundamental aspects of *trans* fats. Chapter 1 is a chemists' view of the *trans* fats problem, the current status and an insight into possible future solutions. Chapter 2 provides the background, scientific basis and the details of new *trans* fats regulation. Chapter 3 discusses the collective summary of *trans* fats clinical trials and the dietary guidelines from various professional health organizations. The second part of the book from chapters 4 to 6 covers the practical aspects of *trans* fats. Chapter 4 evaluates and summarizes the state-of-the-art analytical methods to determine the *trans* fats. Chapter 5 gives an account of the *trans* fat problem, its implications and the potential solutions. Chapter 6 provides insight into the consumer interpretation of the *trans* fats information. The last part, chapter 7 and the Appendix, deal with the commercial aspects of *trans* fats. Chapter 7 is a primer for food product reformulators to consider various practical issues before making the decision on a suitable solution(s). This chapter brings out the importance of various business objectives before reformulation. The Appendix brings the reality of what actual commercial solutions exist to address the *trans* fats in food products. Fats and oils suppliers, such as Aarhus, ADM, Bunge, Cargill, Loders Croklaan, and Premium Vegetable Oils address this issue by providing the actual *trans* fats solutions that they currently offer to their customers.

Bringing this book to reality was a great challenge to contributors, the AOCS staff and us, as it was compiled within a time span of 7 weeks. We greatly appreciate strong commitment and cooperation from all the contributors. Without their unwavering involvement, this book would not have been possible. We express our special thanks to AOCS books, special publications committee members, and its chair for their approval of the project. We gratefully acknowledge the help, guidance and the logistical support from AOCS staff Jodey Schonfeld and Daryl Horrocks, as well as the editorial help from Sithara Kodali.

We hope the information contained in this book helps ease the transition to the new FDA regulations for *trans* fats. We invite readers to contact us and/or any of our contributors with questions or comments to learn more. The readers can find more information about the contributors from the short bio and the contact information provided in the beginning of the book. We hope that this book provides a useful and timely reference in an era of nutritional change in the United States that marks a paradigm shift for fats and oils suppliers worldwide.

Dharma R. Kodali
Gary R. List
March 25, 2005

Contents

Preface   v

Contributors   ix

Chapter 1   *Trans* Fats—Chemistry, Occurrence, Functional Need
in Foods and Potential Solutions
Dharma R. Kodali   1

Chapter 2   *Trans* Fat—New FDA Regulations
Julie Schrimpf-Moss and Virginia Wilkening   26

Chapter 3   Nutritional Considerations of *trans* Fatty Acids
J. Edward Hunter   34

Chapter 4   Determination of *trans* Fats by Gas Chromatography
and Infrared Methods
Magdi Mossoba, John K.G. Kramer, Pierluigi Delmonte,
Martin P. Yurawecz, and Jeanne I. Rader   47

Chapter 5   Dietary Guidelines, Processing, and Reformulation
for *trans* Reduction
G.R. List and Robert Reeves   71

Chapter 6   Communicating with Consumers About *trans* Fat:
The Importance of Consumer Research
Shelley Goldberg, Susan T. Borra, and Diane Quagliani   87

Chapter 7   *Trans* Fat Reformulation Is Not a Technical Objective!
Willie Loh   96

Appendix   Commercial Solutions   106
Aarhus United USA   107
ADM NovaLipids   110
Bunge Oils   114
Cargill Specialty Oils   117
Loders Croklaan   119
Premium Vegetable Oils Sdn Bhd   124

Index   129

CONTRIBUTORS

Susan T. Borra, RD
Executive Vice President
International Food Information Council
1100 Connecticut Ave, NW, Ste 430
Washington DC 20036
borra@ific.org
Susan Borra, RD, a contributor to Chapter 6, is executive vice president at the International Food Information Council (IFIC) in Washington, DC, a nonprofit organization that communicates sound, science-based information on nutrition and food safety to health professionals, educators, government officials, journalists and consumers. Susan directs communications programs, executing public affairs strategies, and managing nutrition and food safety issues. She also oversees the development of consumer education materials and programs about nutrition, food safety and health. IFIC and the IFIC Foundation programs are supported by the food and beverage industry. Susan is active in the American Dietetic Association (ADA), American Heart Association and the Society for Nutrition Education. She also served as a member on the Subcommittee on Interpretation and Uses of Dietary Reference Intakes of the National Academy of Sciences. Susan has a Bachelor's degree in nutrition and dietetics from the University of Maryland, and is a registered dietitian.

Pierluigi Delmonte
Visiting Scientist
U.S. Food and Drug Administration
5100 Pain Branch Pkway
College Park, MD 20740-3835
pierluigi.delmonte@cfsan.fda.gov
Pierluigi Delmonte, a contributor to Chapter 4, is a visiting scientist in the Division of Research and Applied Technology in the Office of Nutritional Products, Labeling and Dietary Supplements.

Shelley Goldberg, MPH, RD
Associate Director, Nutrition Communications
International Food Information Council
1100 Connecticut Ave, NW, Ste 430
Washington DC 20036
Goldberg@ific.org
Shelley Goldberg, a contributor to Chapter 6, is an associate director at the International Food Information Council (IFIC). At IFIC, Shelley is responsible for managing various aspects of nutritionally related programs and initiatives on issues including obesity, carbohydrates and sugars, fats, sodium, and communicating with consumers about nutrition. Prior to joining the IFIC staff, Shelley facilitated committee activities at the National Academy of Science's Food and Nutrition Board on projects including Dietary Reference Intakes and the Role of Dietary Supplements in

Health. She is a member of the ADA, Society for Nutrition Education and the American Council on Exercise. She earned her Bachelors degree at The Pennsylvania State University, her Masters of Public Health degree from the University of Massachusetts at Amherst, and is a registered dietitian.

J. Edward Hunter, Ph.D.
Adjunct Professor
Department of Chemistry
University of Cincinnati
P.O. Box 210172
Cincinnati, OH 45221-0172
hunterje@email.uc.edu
Ed Hunter, author of Chapter 3, is an Adjunct Professor of Chemistry at the University of Cincinnati. He received a B.S. Degree in Chemistry from Lehigh University and M.S. and Ph.D. Degrees in Biochemistry from the University of Wisconsin. After completing his Ph.D. Degree, he joined the Procter & Gamble Company in Cincinnati as a staff scientist. At P&G he provided nutrition support for the Company's food brands, focusing primarily on health effects of dietary fats. He also served as a toxicologist supporting the safety of P&G's hair care brands. After retiring from P&G, he joined the Chemistry Department at the University of Cincinnati as an Adjunct Professor, teaching First-Year Chemistry courses for science and engineering students. In 2002, he received the Dean's Award from UC's College of Arts and Sciences for Distinguished Adjunct Performance. He has published articles and has presented talks at professional meetings on dietary fatty acids in relation to health. In addition, he has done consulting projects for the International Life Sciences Institute, North America, and for the Institute of Shortening and Edible Oils, Inc., both in Washington, D.C.

Bob Johnson
Bunge Oils
725 N. Kinzie Avenue
Bradley, IL 60914
Bob.Johnson@Bunge.com
Bob Johnson, contributor to the Appendix, holds a B.S. in Food Science from Iowa State University, and a M.A. in Food Science from Pennsylvania State University. He joined Bunge aas an R&D Project Leader in 1994 and is presently Team Director of Food Processor R&D. His areas of focus are presently shortenings, margarines, and oils for bakery and food processor applications, and *trans* fatty acid reduction technologies.

Dharma R. Kodali, Ph.D.
Global Agritech Inc.
710 Olive Lane N
Minneapolis, MN 55447
kodali@globalagritech.us
Dharma R. Kodali, book editor and author of Chapter 1, received a Ph. D. in syn-

thetic medicinal chemistry in 1980 from Kurukshetra University. After a year of Post Doctoral training at Polytechnic University in New York, he worked at Boston University for 10 years. As an Assistant Professor of Biophysics he extensively studied structurally defined lipid synthesis, molecular packing, physical properties and their influence on metabolism. As principal scientist and R&D Manager at Cargill for 13 years, he championed new and value-added product development in the areas of biotechnology, food and industrial applications. The research group he led was responsible for the development and commercialization of a number of innovative products. Recently, he was at General Mills as a Corporate Sr. Principal Scientist developing *trans* fat alternatives and as a corporate resource in fats. Currently he is with Global Agritech, a company he established to develop new and value-added bio-products from agricultural materials. Dr. Kodali is a well-recognized expert in lipids and has given numerous invited lectures and presentations in number of international conferences. His accomplishments, among others, include Cargill's Chairman's Innovation Award, the American Chemical Society's Great Lakes Industrial Innovation Award and the AOCS T.L. Mounts award. Dr. Kodali authored/coauthored 60 publications and invented/co-invented 18 patents.

John K.G. Kramer
Agric & Agric Food Canada
Food Research Program
93 Stone Rd W
Guelph, ON N1G 5C9
Canada
kramerj@agr.gc.ca
John K.G. Kramer, a contributor to Chapter 4, is a senior research scientist at the Food Research Program of Agriculture and Agri-Food Canada in Guelph, Ontario, Canada.

Gary List
USDA, NCAUR
Peoria, IL
listgr@ncaur.usda.gov
Gary List, book editor and coauthor of Chapter 5, is a Lead Scientist at the National Center for Agricultural Utilization Research in Peoria, Illinois where he has conducted research on edible fats and oils since 1963. He is the author of over 270 technical publications, abstracts and book chapters including three revisions of the standard fats and oils textbook, "Bailey's Industrial Oil and Fat Products." He has made over 100 presentations at national/international scientific meetings and serves on the editorial boards of three journals. He is a member of AOCS, ACS, IFT, AACC, AAIC, DGF, SCI, and European Federation of Lipids. He is a Fellow in the American Oil Chemists' Society and is the recipient of the AOCS Bailey Medal and the IFT Chang Award for Lipid/Flavor Science.

Willie H. Loh, Ph.D.
Cargill Specialty Canola Oils
P.O. Box 5693/Lake
Minneapolis, MN 55417
willie_loh@cargill.com
Willie Loh, author of Chapter 7 and contributor to the Appendix, is the National Sales Manager for Cargill's Specialty Canola Oils business unit. He heads a team of sales managers responsible for market development and sales of high oleic canola and sunflower oils. Prior to joining Cargill, Willie was the Director of Research & Development for InterMountain Canola Company, a wholly owned subsidiary of DuPont Agricultural Products Group. Willie received his Bachelor's Degree in Biology from Columbia. He also has a Master's Degree in Botany from Rutgers University and a Ph.D. in Microbiology from the Ohio State University. Willie has published original research articles in Oil Chemistry, Oilseed Biochemistry, Microbial Physiology and Plant Molecular Genetics and has been granted more than a dozen patents in these areas. He is an inventor on most of the patents issued for high oleic canola. Cargill's Specialty Canola Oils Business Unit develops, manufactures and markets high oleic oils, primarily canola, to food processing and food service customers in North America.

Mark Matlock
Vice President, Research & Development
Archer Daniels Midland Co.
James R. Randall Res Ctr
1001 N. Brush College Rd
Decatur, IL 62521-1656
Matlock@ADMWORLD.COM
Mark Matlock, contributor to the Appendix, is senior vice president for the ADM Research Division where he directs food ingredient research. Mark joined ADM in 1980 as an analytical chemist and has held positions as manager of process development; laboratory manager of ADM BioProducts; & director of food applications. Mark received a Bachelor of Science degree in chemistry from Millikin University in 1976 and a Master of Science degree in polymer chemistry from the University of Akron in 1987. Mark is author or co-author of seven U.S. patents, two of which relate to an analytical instrument (OSI) that measures the oxidative stability of vegetable oils. He has conducted research that as led to new soy protein isolates for ADM. He has managed research efforts that lead the introduction of trans free fats for margarines and shortenings via a novel enzymatic rearrangement technology. Also, he was elected president of the American Oil Chemists' Society for 2003-2004.

Gerald P. McNeill, Ph.D.
Director Core Products
Loders Croklaan
24708 West Durkee Road,

Channahon, Illinois 60410, USA
gerald.mcneill@croklaan.com
Dr. McNeill, contributor to the Appendix, is currently director of R&D and marketing for core products, Loders Croklaan NA, where he is responsible for introduction of no-trans, non-hydrogenated fat solutions for the food industry. Before joining the Loders operation in 1998, he worked at Unilver Research in England, managing the Loders Croklaan corporate research team. His projects included a discovery program for healthy lipds for the supplement industry, and the development of enzyme technologies for the modification of fats and oils which have been commercialized. Prior to Unilever, Dr. McNeill carried out basic research into enzymatic modification of fats at public institutions, including the USDA in Philadelphia, and Nagoya University, Japan.

Magdi M. Mossoba
FDA Center for Food Safety & Applied Nutrition
5100 Paint Branch Pkway
Rm BE-012
College Park, MD 20740-3835
mmossoba@cfsan.fda.gov
Magdi M. Mossoba, contributor to Chapter 4, is a research chemist at the Office of Scientific Analysis and Support of the U.S. Food and Drug Administration's Center for Food Safety and Applied Nutrition, in College Park, Maryland 20740 USA.

Diane Quagliani, MBA, RD, LDN
Quagliani Communications, Inc.
Specializing in Food, Nutrition and Health
5313 Howard Avenue
Western Springs, IL 60558
dquagliani@aol.com
Registered dietitian Diane Quagliani, a contributor to Chapter 6, is president of Quagliani Communications, Inc., a Chicago-area firm specializing in nutrition communications for consumer and health professional audiences. Diane's consumer nutrition articles have appeared in *Better Homes and Gardens, Weight Watchers Magazine, Teen, American Health for Women,* the *LA Times,* the *Chicago Tribune* and in special interest publications for *Better Homes and Gardens* and *Woman's Day.* She also writes for several Better Homes and Gardens food and health books. Diane has presented on the topic of effective nutrition communications at professional meetings of organizations such as the ADA, the American College of Sports Medicine and the International Congress of Dietetics, as well as at state and local meetings. Her articles have appeared in professional publications such as the *Journal of the American Dietetic Association, Nutrition Today* and *Today's Dietitian.* In addition, she coauthored ADA's 2002 position paper on Food and Nutrition Misinformation. Diane holds a BS degree in dietetics from Bowling Green State University of Ohio, and a BS degree in Psychology and an MBA from Loyola University of Chicago.

Jeanne I. Rader
Director, Division of Research & Applied Technology
Office of Nutritional Products, Labeling and Dietary Supplements
FDA Center for Food Safety & Applied Nutrition
5100 Paint Branch Pkway
Rm BE-012
College Park, MD 20740-3835
jrader@cfsan.fda.gov

Jeanne I. Rader, a contributor to Chapter 4, is the Director, Division of Research and Applied Technology, in the Office of Nutritional Products, Labeling and Dietary Supplements at the U.S. Food and Drug Administration's Center for Food Safety and Applied Nutrition, in College Park, Maryland 20740.

Robert M. Reeves
Institute of Shortening and Edible Oils
1750 New York Ave, NW, Ste 120
Washington, DC 20006
rmreeves@iseo.org

Robert M. Reeves, coauthor of Chapter 5, is President of the Institute of Shortening and Edible Oils, Inc. This trade association represents the interests of the refiners of edible fats and oils who currently process approximately 90–95% of the edible fats and oils in the U.S. He develops policy on issues pertaining to technical matters, the environment, occupational health and safety, energy and government relations.

U.R. Sahasranamam (U.R.S)
President
Premium Vegetable Oils Sdn Bhd
27th Floor, Wisma Tun Sanbandan
Jalan SultanSulaiman
50000, Kuala Lumpur
Malaysia
urs@premium-kl.com

U.R. Sahasranamam, contributor to the Appendix, holds a Bachelors degree in Chemical Engineering (Honours) from the University of Kerala, India; completed a Food Extrusion Module at Colorado State University, USA; a Project Management Course at the Indian Institute of Management, Ahmedabad, India; trained in oil seed processing at Dawson Oil Mills, Minneapolis, USA and Farmland Industries, Kansas, USA. His 33-plus years in the oils and fats industry includes managerial positions at Sundatta Foods and Fibres Ltd., India; M.P. State Oils Seeds Federation, India; Malwa Cotton Seed Products; MP State Coop Oilseed Federation as Project; Britannia Industries Ltd, India (then associate company of Nabisco Brands); Premium Vegetable Oils Sdn. Bhd, where he currently is President of the Premium Sales, Marketing and New Product Development. He has been responsible for developing several *trans* fat alternatives and has several product patents.

Julie Schrimpf-Moss, Ph.D.
U.S. Food and Drug Administration
Center for Food Safety and Applied Nutrition
5100 Paint Branch Parkway
College Park, MD 20740
julie.moss@fda.gov
Dr. Julie Moss, author of Chapter 2, joined the FDA in 2001 as a consumer safety officer in the Center for Food Safety and Applied Nutrition. She began her FDA career in the Office of Plant and Dairy Foods developing policy for the microbiological safety of fresh fruits and vegetables, coordinating and instructing international training courses for produce safety related issues (e.g., good agricultural practices), and assisting in the development of FDA's bioterrorism regulations. Presently, Dr. Moss is in the Office of Nutritional Products, Labeling and Dietary Supplements and is involved in nutrition policy for trans fat, health claims, and nutrition labeling. Dr. Moss holds a bachelor's degree in medical nutrition from The Ohio State University, a master's degree in nutrition from the University of Cincinnati and a doctorate in food science from the Florida State University.

Virginia Wilkening
20 W. Linden St.
Alexandria, VA 22301
cvmbw@yahoo.com
Virginia Wilkening, coauthor of Chapter 2, retired in April 2004 from the position of Deputy Director, Office of Nutritional Products, Labeling, and Dietary Supplements (ONPLDS) in the Center for Food Safety and Applied Nutrition (CFSAN), Food and Drug Administration (FDA). As Deputy Director, Ms. Wilkening shared responsibility for developing policy and regulations for dietary supplements, nutrition labeling, food standards, infant formula and medical foods as well as for compliance/enforcement actions and scientific evaluation to support such regulations and related policy development, and analytical database research. Ms. Wilkening earned her Master of Science degree in nutrition at the University of California in Davis, California. She attended a dietetic internship at Grasslands Hospital (now part of New York Medical Center) in Valhalla, New York. Her Bachelor of Science degree is also from the University of California at Davis with a major in nutrition and dietetics.

Ed Wilson
Sales & Marketing Director
Aarhus United USA
973-344-1300
ed.wilson@aarhusunited.com
Currently Sales & Marketing Director for Aarhus United USA Inc., **Ed Wilson** worked in Technical Service and R&D, focusing on the confectionery and baking industries. He majored in industrial management while attending The College of Philadelphia and Glassboro State University; and has participated in many short courses sponsored by

universities and trade organizations. He is active in the following associations, A.A.C.T., P.M.C.A., A.O.C.S. and the IFT.

Martin P. Yurawecz
U.S. Food and Drug Administration
5100 Paint Branch Pkway
Ste HFS-840, Rm 1E009
College Park, MD 20740-3835
mpy@cfsan.fda.gov
Martin P. Yurawecz, contributor to Chapter 4, is a research chemist in the Division of Research and Applied Technology in the Office of Nutritional Products, Labeling and Dietary Supplements.

Chapter 1

Trans Fats—Chemistry, Occurrence, Functional Need in Foods and Potential Solutions

Dharma R. Kodali

Global Agritech Inc., 710 Olive Ln. N., Minneapolis, MN 55447-4203; kodali@globalagritech.us

Introduction

Natural oils and fats are liquids or semisolids consisting primarily of triacylglycerols (TAG). In literature, TAG are often referred to as triglycerides, even though this latter term is less accurate in representing the molecular structure of this class of compounds. The distinction between fats and oils is seen by their physical state at ambient temperature; the fats are solid and the oils are liquid. The two major sources of oils and fats are from animals and plants. Greater than 90% of commercial oils and fats used for human consumption are plant-derived vegetable oils. Unrefined natural oils and fats, after extraction from the source, comprise mostly TAG containing less than 5% of minor components such as sterols, phospholipids, tocopherols, fatty acids and partial glycerol esters. The minor components and their concentration in the crude oil depend upon the origin and method of oil extraction. The crude oils are subjected to various processing steps like degumming and alkali refining (to remove phospholipids and fatty acids), bleaching (to remove colored and polar matter) and steam stripping or deodorization (to remove volatile components) to make them suitable for human consumption. Oils subjected to these steps are usually referred to as RBD (refined, bleached and deodorized) oils and contain about 99% TAG.

The major vegetable oils of commerce are soybean, cottonseed, canola, sunflower, corn, peanut, palm, palm kernel and coconut oils. Other vegetable oils like olive, rice bran, safflower, sesame and other specialty oils are not used extensively due to availability and cost. A typical chemical structure of TAG is shown in Figure 1.1. The TAG contains a glycerol backbone with three hydroxyls esterified to three long linear carboxylic acids called fatty acids. The glycerol portion of TAG is constant in all oils and fats. The type of fatty acid structure and the position of esterification on glycerol differ from one TAG to another. Glycerol is a prochiral molecule capable of forming two different TAG stereoisomers when esterified with different fatty acid chains at the 1- and 3-positions. These stereoisomers when differentiated from one another are identified as stereospecifically numbered, -*sn*-glycerol derivatives (Kodali *et al.*, 1984, 1989a). Even though biological systems can recognize the isomeric -*sn*-glycerol derivatives, the physical and chemical properties of these isomers are very similar. For all functional and practical purposes they are treated as one and the same.

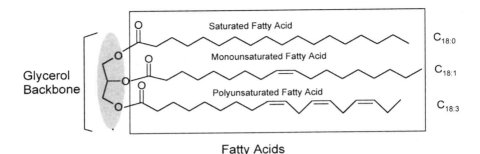

Fatty Acids

Fig. 1.1. A typical molecular structure of a triacylglycerol showing the glycerol backbone region esterified with three different fatty acids: stearic, oleic, and linolenic acids.

Vegetable oils contain a mixture of specific TAG molecules of given concentrations. Fatty acid structures differ from each other in carbon chain length and the number of double bonds. Most of the naturally occurring fatty acids are even numbered, 4 to 24 carbon atoms long. They are synthesized by the biological systems from two-carbon unit acetyl coenzyme A. More prevalent saturated fatty acids with no double bonds that occur in oils and fats are lauric (C_{12}), myristic (C_{14}), palmitic (C_{16}) and stearic (C_{18}) acids. The number in the parenthesis shows the number of carbon atoms corresponding to the fatty acid chain length. Sometimes a zero after the number indicates that there are no double bonds. The predominant unsaturated fatty acids are oleic ($C_{18:1}$), linoleic ($C_{18:2}$) and linolenic ($C_{18:3}$) acids. The numbers in the parenthesis show the carbon chain length followed by the number of double bonds. The position of double bonds in the chain and the double bond configuration are also very important. In oleic acid it is at carbon-9, in linoleic at 9 and 12 and in linolenic at 9, 12 and 15. Most of the unsaturated fatty acids that occur in natural fats and oils –with few exceptions, have the double bonds in *cis* configuration. The fatty acids that contain a single double bond are referred to as "monounsaturated" and others with more than one double bond are "polyunsaturated" fatty acids. Even though there are hundreds of different fatty acids that occur in oils and fats, the fatty acids referred above are most common and abundant in natural oils and fats.

The predominant vegetable oils in commerce can be divided into three types based on carbon chain length—lauric, palmitic and oleic oils. The lauric oils, mostly coconut and palm kernel oils, contain high levels of 12-carbon lauric acid. The common palmitic oil, palm oil, contains 16-carbon palmitic acid in high concentration. The lauric and palmitic oils are high in saturated fatty acids and are semisolids at ambient temperature. Because coconut, palm and palm kernel oils are grown in the temperate regions, they are referred to as tropical oils. Oleic oils predominantly contain 18- carbon fatty acids, stearic, oleic, linoleic and linolenic acids. The soybean, cottonseed, canola, corn and peanut oils belong in this category. The major types of edible oils that are consumed in North America are soybean, corn and canola. Palm oil is not extensively used in the United States but is more common in Asia and

Europe. Soybean and palm are the two most abundantly available vegetable oils in the world, each accounting for close to 25% of the total worldwide oils and fats production of about 120 million tons/year.

Defining vegetable oil composition by individual TAG structure and concentration is more accurate but very cumbersome. This requires sophisticated methodology in separating and identifying the various TAG species. Because of this reason, vegetable oils are identified by gross fatty acid composition (by weight). The fatty acid composition of most edible oils in commerce is shown in Table 1.1. The fatty acid composition of various vegetable oils is determined by plant variety and genetics. In a given variety the fatty acid composition changes a little, due to geography and environmental factors. Because of this variation the fatty acid composition is often expressed as a range rather than a single number. The fatty acid compositions given in Table 1.1 are given in average weight percent.

Recent developments in biotechnology and plant breeding make it possible to develop new genetic varieties, which yield oils with different fatty acid composition than traditional oils. For example, the oil from regular canola is composed of 62% oleic acid whereas the high oleic and very high oleic canola varieties are composed of about 75 and 84% oleic acid, respectively.

There are numerous review articles that deal with composition, processing, physical and chemical properties and commercial aspects of oils and fats (Technical committee of the ISEO, 1994; Hasenhuettl 1994, Thomas 2003). More comprehensive and detailed information is provided in Bailey's (Bailey's 1996). Another source of chemical and physical property information on various specific fatty acids, TAG, partial glycerol esters is provided in The Lipid Handbook (Gunstone *et al.*, 1994).

TABLE 1.1
The Fatty Acid Composition (wt.%) of Conventional and High Oleic Oils

Oil Type	S.C.[a] C6–10	Lauric C12	Myristic C14	Palmitic C16	Stearic C18	L.C.[b] C20–24	Oleic C18:1	Linoleic C18:2	Linolenic C18:3
Soybean	—	—	—	11	4	—	23	55	7
Cottonseed	—	—	1	22	3	—	19	54	1
Sunflower	—	—	—	7	5	—	19	68	1
Canola	—	—	—	4	2	—	62	22	10
H. Oleic Canola	—	—	—	4	2	2	75	12	5
VHO[c] Canola	—	—	—	4	2	1	84	5	4
Peanut	—	—	—	11	2	7	48	32	—
Corn	—	—	—	11	2	—	28	58	1
Coconut	15	47	18	9	3	—	6	2	—
Palm kernel	8	48	16	8	2	—	15	3	—
Palm	—	—	1	45	4	—	40	10	—

[a]Short Chain C-6 hexanoic (caproic), C-8 octanoic (caprylic), C-10 decanoic (Capric) fatty acids.
[b]Long Chain C-20 Eicosanoic (arachidic), C-22 docosanoic (behenic), C-24 tetracosanoic (lignoceric) fatty acids.
[c]Very High Oleic.

Cis, Trans Isomerism

The double bond present in the fatty acid inhibits the rotation of carbons on either side and thereby fixes the configuration of atoms present on double bond carbons. Because of this fixed geometry the hydrogen atoms present on double bond carbons can be on the same side (*cis,* in Latin) or on the opposite side (*trans,* in Latin). The "*cis*" and "*trans*" are written in *italics* to identify their Latin origin and to represent the chemical configuration as shown in Figure 1.2. *Cis* and *trans* isomers are geometric isomers as they differ from one another only in the way that the atoms are oriented in space. The double bond is rigid and creates a kink in the chain. The rest of the chain is free to rotate about the other C-C single bonds. In general *trans* compounds have higher melting points than the corresponding *cis* isomers, reflecting the greater ease of crystal packing of the somewhat more symmetrical molecules. The interconversion of *cis* and *trans* takes place by the breaking and reformation of the double bond, which requires about 65kcal/mole of energy. Because of this high energy barrier the *cis* and *trans* isomerization does not occur easily, unless assisted by a catalyst or high temperatures.

The *cis* isomer is more asymmetric than the corresponding *trans* isomer and cannot pack well into a crystal lattice. Because of this reason the *trans* isomers have a higher density, lower solubility and a higher melting point. *Trans* isomers are less sterically hindered and more thermodynamically stable than *cis*. Therefore, the *cis* isomer can be transformed into a *trans* isomer by subjecting it to a high temperature. Very high temperatures provide enough energy to cause rotation about the double bond to convert *cis* configuration into a more stable *trans* isomer, an irreversible process. During vegetable oil refining, the oil is subjected to steam deodorization to remove the volatile compounds. The high temperature conditions of deodorization cause *trans* isomerization. Because of this reason most of the refined oils—even though not subjected to hydrogenation—contain as much as 1-2% of *trans* fats.

Functional Need for Solid Fat in Food Products

The oils/fats, besides proteins and carbohydrates are one of the three major classes of building blocks required for living organisms. They are the most concentrated form of energy (9 cal/gram) and because of this most living organisms use them as an

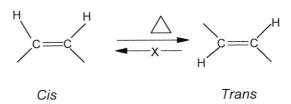

Cis   Trans

Fig. 1.2. *Cis, trans* isomerism of a double bond under thermal conditions.

energy storage medium. In various food applications oils and fats provide a number of functional benefits. They provide lubricity, decrease the interfacial tension of food particles thereby making the food more palatable and easier to swallow. They supply essential fatty acids and oil-soluble vitamins that are essential for various biological functions.

The chemical composition of a mixture of TAG molecules present in a given vegetable oil is responsible for its physical state at ambient temperature. The oils containing saturated fatty acids in high concentration, like coconut and palm, can provide unique functionality and are more oxidatively stable. In general, the physical state of liquid (oil) or solid (fat) can possess some general and specific characteristics as is shown in Table 1.2.

There are two primary reasons to use fats instead of oils—oxidative stability and solid fat functionality. These properties are very important depending upon the food application. In some frying applications, like snacks, the oxidative stability is very important but the solid fat content (SFC) is not. In baking applications, both of these properties are important. Lack of sufficient oxidative stability affects the shelf life of the food product. Oxidation is the cause of off-flavors and rancidity.

Solid fats can be preferred in food applications because they are resistant to oxidation. In oxidation, vegetable oils react with molecular oxygen to form hydroperoxides, which in turn break down to create radicals that promote further oxidation. The break-down products formed during oxidation lead to off-flavors. The ease of oxidation depends upon the fatty acid structure. The saturated fatty acids are much more stable than unsaturated fatty acids. The rate of oxidation of monounsaturated oleic acid is about 10 times greater than saturated stearic acid. The polyunsaturated linoleic acid undergoes oxidation 10 times faster than oleic and half as fast as linolenic acid (Kodali 2003a). The oxidation rates indicate that saturated fats are more stable than unsaturated fats and will have a longer shelf life. The oil containing polyunsaturated fatty acids are much more susceptible to oxidation than oils containing monounsaturated fatty acids. For this reason the low linolenic and high oleic oils have better functionality for frying applications. The oxidative stability of oils and fats affects the shelf life, process life, and the flavor of a food product.

The hardness of a fat imparts certain desirable properties such as crispiness, snap, and texture to a food product. The fats that are used in food applications contain a mixture of TAG. The composition and individual TAG chemical structure of a fat determines how much will be liquid and solid at room temperature. In fats,

TABLE 1.2
General Properties of Oils and Fats

Functional property	Oils (liquids)	Fats (solids)
Oxidative stability	Low	High
Hardness	None	Texture, spreadability, snap
Mouth feel	Good	Better

liquid oil is entrapped in a solid matrix, giving a solid or semisolid appearance. The percentage of solid fat in a fat matrix is quantified by the solid fat index (SFI) or the solid fat content (SFC). SFI measures the change in volume with temperature. The liquids have higher volume than solids; the volume decreases with the increase in degree of crystallinity within solids. SFC is measured by nuclear magnetic resonance that takes advantage of molecular mobility as indicated by signal broadening. The molecular mobility of liquids decreases as the crystallinity (SFC) increases, which broadens the signal. The results of SFI and SFC do not correlate well but both measure the percentage of solid fat with the change in temperature. This information is very useful in assessing the functionality of a fat in a given application.

In some formulations a certain amount of solid fat is necessary to entrap the liquid oil to prevent oiling-off. In retail popcorn packaging, for example, oiling-off discolors the packaging, giving the consumer a perception of damaged goods. The hardness of fat also provides brittleness or a snap in products like chocolates. If a sufficient amount of solid fat of the formulation melts much above the body temperature of 37°C, it leaves an undesirable waxy coating in the mouth. Because of this reason, solid fats that melt above 40°C are not used in higher concentration in food product formulations. On the other hand, if a solid fat has a very high amount of solids at room temperature and melts very quickly at or below body temperature, it creates a smooth cooling sensation in the mouth as it absorbs the energy from the mouth cavity. The cooling sensation is proportional to the enthalpy of melting. Therefore the fats with higher enthalpy will have the greater effect. The melting of the fat also releases other ingredients responsible for taste and flavor, giving a burst of euphoric sensation.

Cocoa butter is an excellent example to demonstrate the desirable properties of solid fat. Cocoa butter is more homogeneous in composition than most natural fats, with only three fatty acids—palmitic, stearic and oleic—constituting more than 95% of the composition. The three fatty acids, found in high concentration, lead to the formation of few TAG structures. This relative structural homogeneity and high amount of saturates provide cocoa butter fat with both high melting temperature and stability. The ratio of saturated to unsaturated fatty acids is 2:1; when combined with nature's propensity to attach unsaturated fatty acids at the 2-position of glycerol, symmetrical TAG structures like POP and SOS are favored. In general, symmetrical TAG have higher melting temperatures than their unsymmetrical counterparts. The high melting temperature and steep melting curve of cocoa butter can be observed by measuring the SFC of cocoa butter with temperature as shown in Figure 1.3.

Cocoa butter has a very high SFC at or below room temperature (Figure 1.3). Because of this, products containing high concentrations of cocoa butter have good dimensional stability and a snap to the bite. Once in the mouth cavity the fat melts rapidly by absorbing the surrounding energy. The sharp melting between 20 to 35°C and high enthalpy gives cocoa butter unique and valuable properties that demonstrate the importance of solid fat in food.

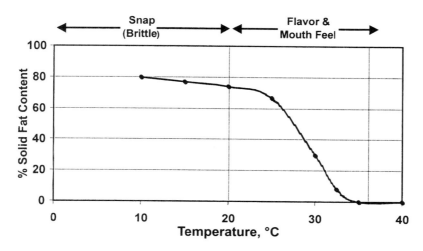

Fig. 1.3. Cocoa butter melting behavior, change in solid fat content with temperature.

Properties and Source of *Trans*

The unsaturated fatty acids present in the natural oils and fats are in *cis* configuration. The *cis* isomers are relatively asymmetric and pack poorly in the crystal lattice due to a kink in the middle of the hydrocarbon chain. This kink in the middle of the chain reduces the inter-chain interactions in the solid state, thereby lowering the melting temperature and enthalpy. Compared to *cis* double bonds, *trans* double bonds are relatively symmetric and pack better in the crystal lattice, so their melting temperature falls between the melting temperatures of saturated and *cis* unsaturated fatty acids. A comparison of the molecular structures and melting temperatures of three fatty acids of 18-carbon chain length, oleic acid (*cis*-9 double bond), elaidic acid (*trans*-9 double bond), and stearic acid illustrate this point. The molecular structures with space filling models and melting temperatures are shown in Figure 1.4.

Nature utilized the *cis* configuration to make the high molecular weight TAG molecules as large as 900 Daltons and still keep them in the liquid state at ambient temperature. Biological processes occur more efficiently and molecules are more accessible in a liquid state. Because of this the fatty acid composition of various vegetable oils reflect the climatic and geographic conditions. Tropical oils contain saturated fatty acids in higher concentration whereas the oleic oils that are grown in a colder climate contain polyunsaturated fatty acids in greater concentration.

Soybean oil is the most abundant vegetable oil worldwide, accounting for 25% of the total world production. It is also the most-consumed vegetable oil in the United States. Soybean oil is composed of more than 60% polyunsaturated fatty acids, which react readily with oxygen to form hydroperoxides. To improve the oxidative stability by reducing the content of polyunsaturated fatty acids of soybean

D.R. Kodali

Stearic Acid MP 70°C

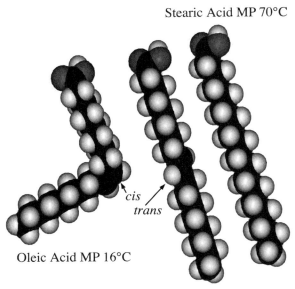

Oleic Acid MP 16°C

Elaidic Acid MP 44°C

Fig. 1.4. The molecular structures of oleic acid (*cis*-9, m.p. 16°C), elaidic acid (*trans*-9, m.p. 44°C) and stearic acid (m.p. 70°C).

oil, hydrogenation was invented in the early 20th century. Partial hydrogenation of vegetable oils is the major source of *trans* fats in food products. The *trans* fat content of hydrogenated fats varies from 10% to as much as 40% based upon the extent of hydrogenation and hydrogenation conditions. This will be further discussed in the hydrogenation process described below. Minor amounts of *trans* fats also form under the deodorization conditions of vegetable oil processing. Another source of *trans* fats is of animal origin from dairy and meat products. The concentration of *trans* fats in dairy and meat fats is usually low, from 3-8%, and these *trans* fats are different from those formed by hydrogenation of vegetable oils. The bacteria present in the ruminants' gut hydrolyses the dietary fat and subjects the resulting fatty acids to biohydrogenation. The initial step in this process involves the conversion of *cis*-12 double bond in polyunsaturated fatty acids to a *trans*-11 configuration, followed by the hydrogenation of a *cis*-9 double bond. Thus in biohydrogenation process linoleic acid gives rise to vaccinic acid, a *trans*-11 fatty acid. Because of this reason the *trans* fats of animal origin contain *trans*-11 vaccinic acid in greater concentration whereas the partially hydrogenated vegetable oils contain a higher concentration of *trans*-9 elaidic acid (Mossoba *et al.* 2003). The concentration of various *trans* isomers and their relative ratios can help to determine the origin of *trans* fats in the diet. For instance the examination of adipose fat can reveal the source of dietary *trans* fats, from either partially hydrogenated vegetable oil or ruminant fats (Combe 2003).

Trans Fats Reduction/Elimination Technologies

In July 2003, FDA issued a final rule requiring a mandatory declaration in the nutritional label of the amount of *trans* fat present in foods including dietary supplements. The declaration of *trans* fat is to be expressed as grams per serving to the nearest 0.5 gram increment below 5 grams and to the nearest gram increment above 5 grams (Moss and Wilkening 2005). The *trans* fat regulations that will be effective from January 1, 2006 are influencing food product manufacturers either to eliminate or reduce the *trans* fat from their products.

Many fat and oil applications do not require SFC. Most of these applications include deep-frying where thermal and oxidative stabilities are more important. There are some exceptions to this, such as donut frying where the SFC is necessary to provide glaze and crispiness. For frying applications, good oxidative stability can be obtained by using monounsaturated oils, low linolenic oils or formulating with antioxidants. In other applications, like baked goods, a certain amount of SFC is crucial. The solid fats provide the pliability to dough and also give layer, spread or discrete distribution of fat depending upon the product requirement. Some of the unique properties provided by solid fats in baked goods are flakiness, hardness, volume increase, layer separation, air entrapment while baking, dimensional structure and freshness.

There are five core strategic technologies that have the ability to reduce or eliminate the *trans* fat content in foods. These are formulation, modification of fatty acid composition through genetics, hydrogenation, fractionation and interesterification. These are enabling technologies that can be used alone or in combination with each other to create *trans* fat solutions. These technologies and their limitations are discussed below.

Formulation

There are a number of *trans* fat solutions that can be created through formulation (Walter 2004). These strategies include:
  (i) Entrapment of liquid oils. The liquid oils can be entrapped in solid fat matrix. A small percentage of completely hydrogenated soybean oil can entrap a large amount of liquid oil. Care must be taken not to use large amounts of very high melting fats as they can leave a coating in the mouth cavity and create waxiness. Based on the food product formulation, the entrapment can also be achieved by other components present in the formulation, such as emulsifiers.
 (ii) Blending partially hydrogenated fat with stable high oleic oils can provide structure and oxidative stability with reduced *trans* fat content.
(iii) Addition of antioxidants to fats and oils can provide oxidative stability and improve the shelf life of the products. The antioxidants can be natural (such as tocopherols), synthetic, or a combination of both.
(iv) Use of palm fractions can provide the desired SFC without the use of *trans* or hydrogenated fat on the label. However the trade-off comes from the presence of

palm on the label, indicating the use of saturated tropical oil. Formulation with animal fats and their fractions create a similar conundrum of incorporating higher saturates and cholesterol content on the label.

(v) Special hydrogenation conditions can provide low *trans* base stocks that can still permit the "*trans* fat 0g" label depending upon the fat content and serving size as described in the hydrogenation section below.

Genetics

Plant genetics can be modified through conventional plant breeding or genetic engineering. In the past two decades both these techniques have been used to change oilseed bearing plants to modify their fatty acid composition. This process will drastically increase in the next decade to produce various varieties of specialty oils that provide specific functionality for food and industrial applications (Kodali *et al.*, 2003). In a single crop variety there are a number of genotypes which give a specific trait responsible for a specific fatty acid composition. In soybeans, genotypes with special traits have been developed that include low-linolenic, high-oleic, low-palmitic, low-saturate, high-palmitic and high-stearic (Liu 1999). Other varieties target enhancement of levels of minor components such as specific tocopherols. A number of high oleic oils, including canola, sunflower, and safflower, are currently available on the market (Loh 2000). Genetic modification is also targeted towards the creation of high saturated fatty acid varieties that can replace hydrogenated oils with naturally produced solid fats. These fats could be further fractionated to give value-added cocoa butter substitutes (Kodali 2004). Most of these crops are in the developmental stage, and some have to overcome penalties like yield lag to become economically successful.

Hydrogenation

The two primary reasons for hydrogenation are to improve the oxidative stability and to increase the SFC. The improved oxidative stability also improves the flavor and shelf life of the products. The increased SFC increases the melting temperature and provides improved food texture and functionality.

In the hydrogenation process, hydrogen atoms are added to the unsaturated (double) bonds thereby converting them into saturated C-C (single) bonds. The level of unsaturation of oil is measured by the absorption of iodine and expressed as iodine value (IV). During partial hydrogenation, the iodine value of soybean oil is reduced from the initial 126 to a desired IV of 110 to 70 depending upon the required functional properties of the hydrogenated base stock. The hydrogenation is done in the presence of a metal catalyst and pressurized hydrogen gas at high temperature. Even though the addition of hydrogen to the double bonds is the primary reaction during the hydrogenation, other side reactions occur, such as isomerization of double bonds from *cis* to more stable *trans* configuration and migration of the double bonds along the chain (shifting the position of the double bonds in the chain). With the current hydrogenation technology the *trans* formation can be reduced but not eliminated.

Trans formation increases with hydrogenation temperature but decreases with an increase in pressure, catalyst concentration and agitation. Hydrogen starvation during hydrogenation and using a reused or poisoned catalyst can also increase the *trans* formation (Mounts 1987).

Evans *et al.* studied *trans* formation under selective and nonselective conditions of hydrogenation (Evans *et al.*, 1964). The catalyst concentration (0.2%) and the agitation (1380 rpm) were kept the same for both reaction conditions. The hydrogenation conditions employed were selective (170°C), hydrogen pressure (5 psi); nonselective (120°C), hydrogen pressure (100 psi). Under these conditions the measured *trans* formation was about 0.7% per IV unit reduction under selective conditions and 0.4% per IV unit for nonselective conditions. This demonstrates that *trans* formation can be influenced by hydrogenation conditions. However, the saturated content increased more under nonselective conditions than under selective conditions. The type and nature of catalyst also influences the *trans* formation considerably. A typical representation of *trans* and saturates formation during the hydrogenation process is shown in Figure 1.5.

Even though the hydrogenation increases the *trans* and saturates, by manipulating the hydrogenation conditions their formation can be minimized. The temperature and type of catalyst play a big role in *trans* and saturated fat formation (Ariaansz and Okonek 1998). Recently Beers and Mangus reported on low *trans* hydrogenation processes. (Beers and Mangus 2004). *Trans* fat regulations allow "*trans* fat 0g" on the food product label if the product contains below 0.5 g of *trans* fat per serving.

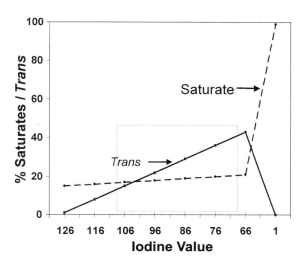

Fig. 1.5. A schematic representation of formation of saturates and *trans* fats of soybean oil during hydrogenation from iodine value of 126 to completely hydrogenated soybean oil of iodine value 2. Most of the hydrogenated base stocks (IV, 110-70) used in food products are shown in the box.

Therefore the *trans* fat content in the fat ingredient, the serving size and the amount of fat used in the food product formulation can determine the ability to use the "*trans* fat 0g" label. The amount of fat allowed per serving in order to use the "*trans* fat 0g" label, based on *trans* fat content is shown in Table 1.3. Many food products contain 3–5 grams of fat/serving. Modification of various hydrogenation conditions and their optimization can lead to low *trans* hydrogenated fats with reasonable functionality (List and King, 2005).

Fractionation

The process of crystallization and separation of low melting liquid and high melting solid portions of a fat mixture is called fractionation. Fractionation can be done with the help of a solvent or without a solvent (dry fractionation). Solvent fractionation done with acetone or hexane is more efficient and gives a cleaner separation of the fractions. Due to greater capital and processing cost involved however, it is seldom practiced. The dry fractionation process is extensively practiced in the palm oil industry (Pantzaris, 2000). The solids and liquids thus separated are called *stearins* and *oleins,* respectively. To make this a viable process certain amounts of solids are necessary at ambient temperatures. Because of this reason, the high saturated or hydrogenated *trans* fatty acid containing oils are good starting feed materials for fractionation. Palm oil is also well suited for fractionation due to its high-saturated fatty acid content. The palm fractions are natural and do not contain *trans* fats. Usually the crystallization is effected by cooling the palm oil very slowly to facilitate the nucleation and growth of a desired crystal structure, morphology and size. The slurry of liquids and solids thus formed are separated by centrifugation or by filtration through a mechanical press by applying pressure. The fractionation process has become very handy in creating different varieties of palm products from very low melting super *oleins* to very high melting hard *stearins* from a single source. A typical palm fractionation process with different fractions and their melting ranges are given in Figure 1.6.

TABLE 1.3
The *trans* Fat Content in the Ingredient and the Corresponding
Amount of Fat/Serving to Allow the Use of "*trans* fat 0 g" on a
Food Product Label

Trans Fat Content (wt%) in the Ingredient	Amount of fat/serving in the formulation (g)
1	49
2	24
3.5	12
7.5	6
15	3
32	1.5
40	1

Palm Oil Fractionation

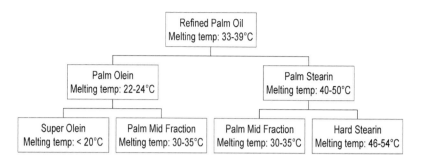

Fig. 1.6. Dry fractionation of palm oil into stearines and oleins.

A typical fatty acid composition of palm oil and palm fractions is shown in Table 1.4. By varying the crystallization temperature, cooling rate and amount of pressure applied during the filtration, a number of palm fractions of different composition and properties can be produced. More than 20 different palm oil fractions are available commercially.

Similar fractional crystallization and filtration is also used on oils that contain small amounts of high melting TAG or waxes. This fractionation is usually called winterization. Winterization is mostly done to remove the turbidity caused by the high melting crystals and to improve the oil clarity at room temperature.

Interesterification

In vegetable oils and fats the distribution of fatty acids on the glycerol backbone is not random. The saturated fatty acids are preferentially esterified to the glycerol primary hydroxyls, 1 and 3, and the unsaturated fatty acids are esterified to the 2-position. The interesterification process is used to modify the distribution of fatty acids, thus modifying the properties of natural or hydrogenated or fractionated oils or fats. Interesterification is a transesterification of two or more oils or fats where the fatty acid arrangement on the glycerol back bone of each of the original TAG is

TABLE 1.4
Typical Fatty Acid Composition of Palm Oil and Palm Fractions

Fatty Acid	Palm Oil	Palm Olein	Superolein	Hard Stearin
Myristic (C14:0)	1	1	1	1.5
Palmitic (C16:0)	47	40	35	60
Stearic (C18:0)	4	4	4	4.5
Oleic (C18:1)	41	43	46	28
Linoleic (C18:2)	11	12	14	6
Melting temp.	33–39°C	20–24°C	15°C	46–54°C

rearranged. Interesterification is done under chemical or enzymatic conditions. In chemical interesterification the distribution of fatty acids on the glycerol backbone of the product is rearranged as per the statistical probability at equilibrium. However, in the enzymatic processes the enzymes are more specific, favoring rearrangement of the fatty acids present at the 1 and 3 positions of glycerol, leaving the 2-position intact. The enzymatic process is commercially applied to produce more exotic fats like cocoa butter substitutes. At present the chemical interesterification process is simpler and more cost effective than the enzymatic process. It is quite possible however, that the enzymatic process could be more cost effective and beneficial in producing the structured TAG of higher value.

The chemical interesterification of two different base stocks with different melting temperatures that produce an intermediate melting product is shown in Figure 1.7. This process can be affected by heating the transesterified components in the presence of a small amount of base catalyst like sodium methoxide. As shown in Figure 1.7, two different fats and oils of different TAG composition and properties can be transesterified to yield an end product of an entirely different composition. The desired physical properties of the end product can be achieved by choosing the composition and the ratio of saturated and unsaturated components. Sometimes the random distribution of fatty acids can be altered by crystallization and separation of higher melting saturated product from the reaction by conducting the transesterification process at temperatures below the crystallization temperature of the high-melting components that form during the reaction. This type of interesterification is called directed transesterification.

Specifically, random chemical transesterification process can be accomplished by drying the base stock to be interesterified at about 100°C under a vacuum, and then adding a base catalyst of about 0.1 wt% to the heated oil. After the catalyst addition, the oil is kept under a vacuum and agitation for 30 minutes to complete the interesterification process. The catalyst can be deactivated by adding bleaching earth and filtration, or by a water wash. The oil thus obtained is dried, bleached and deodorized to produce the final product. Even though the process is simple, care should be taken to prepare the starting oils, as the quality of the feedstock greatly

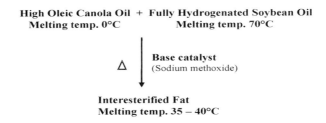

Fig. 1.7. Chemical transesterification of high oleic oil with fully hydrogenated soybean oil gives an interesterified product of intermediate melting temperature.

affects the oil losses. The presence of moisture, fatty acids or peroxides in the feed-stock can kill the catalyst and reduce product yield. Starting feedstock of good quality will require lower amount of catalyst and result in lower oil losses.

Functional Fat with Nutrition/Health Characteristics

It would be useful to find a solid fat that has ideal functional and nutritional characteristics. The new FDA regulations to label the *trans* fats and the resulting consumer perception encourage the elimination or reduction of *trans* fats from food products. The functional void created by the elimination of *trans* can be filled by saturated fats. However, this is not a clean option, as the saturated fats are not considered healthy. Various health organizations recommend that the amount of total dietary fat intake is 30% of the total daily calories. The recommended saturated fat intake should be less than 10% of the daily energy. This translates to one saturated fatty acid per TAG molecule in the fat. At the same time, the fat should provide the right functional properties like hardness at room temperature and high and sharp melting characteristics between 20 and 35°C with high enthalpy of melting. Designing such a functional fat requires an in-depth understanding of the structure-properties-functionality relationship. The discussion of various groups of structurally related pure TAG compounds in the following section will facilitate the concept of such a designer fat.

Designer Fats

Molecular Packing and Polymorphism

The physical properties of a fat depend upon the TAG composition and chemical structure. Therefore, to relate the physical properties of a fat to the functionality, it is crucial to understand the connection between the TAG structure and its influence on the molecular packing. A specific TAG structure and the resulting physical properties have implications in some physiological processes, such as accessibility in aggregated particles like chylomicrons, enzymatic hydrolysis and the subsequent metabolism (Redgrave *et al.*, 1988; Small 1984). Once a fat structure that meets all the functional requirements is identified, it could be produced using the enabling technologies discussed above.

Fats additionally have the propensity to pack in several different crystal structures of comparable lattice energy with different melting temperatures and molecular packing. These different solid-state structures of the same chemical composition are called polymorphs and the phenomenon is called polymorphism. Polymorphism of fats and oils has been well studied and characterized by various techniques like x-ray diffraction and vibrational spectroscopy by different researchers for over 50 years (Chapman 1962; Larson 1964, Kodali *et al.*, 1989a, Sato 1996). Three distinct polymorphic forms, α, β', and β have been characterized based on their hydrocarbon chain packing. In general, α is the least stable and lowest melting polymorphic form with no specific chain-chain interaction, followed by intermediate melting β' with specific chain-chain interaction. The most stable and high melting polymorph is β with very specific molecular packing. These polymorphs are distinguished from each other based on the x-ray diffraction short spacings that characterize the molecular packing on the short axis, called the hydrocarbon sub-cell packing. In reality most of the fats may have more than three polymorphic forms. For example a single TAG structure, 1,2-dipalmitoyl-3-decanoyl-*sn*-glycerol, has been shown to form 5 distinct polymorphs that differ from each other in the molecular packing in the short as well as long axis, resulting in distinct physical properties (Kodali *et al.*, 1989b).

The main factors that contribute to different modes of packing in each polymorphic form are the geometry of the glycerol backbone and the packing of the long hydrocarbon chains along their long and short axis. The packing along the acyl chain length can be identified from the X-ray long spacings, which is also called layered packing. Fatty acid chain length, the presence of one or more double bonds and the position of substitution on the glycerol backbone all influence the layered packing (Kodali *et al.*, 1987, 1989a, 1990).

The molecular structure influences the solid-state behavior of fats with temperature as well as the rates of crystallization and crystal morphology. The understanding of crystal structure, stability and rates of transformation from one polymorphic form to another can relate to some of the gross functional properties. For instance, the discoloration or blooming in chocolates is due to transformation of desirable β-crystal form into another higher melting β-form. In margarines and shortenings, crystallization of β-polymorphic form instead of the desirable β'-polymorph results in large crystal size and morphology responsible for graininess or a sandy feeling in the mouth.

The β' crystals, due to their relatively small crystal size, feel smooth and melt quickly in mouth. It is known in the industry that oils containing higher concentrations of palmitic acid like cottonseed oil stabilize the β'-polymorphic form. For this reason cottonseed oil is added to soybean oil base stocks that are used to make shortenings and margarines. The mismatch of C16 and C18 chain lengths create a methyl end chain packing that stabilizes the β'-polymorphic form. The most stable crystal form in one of the pure TAG with dissimilar chain lengths, 1,2-dipalmitoyl-3-myristoyl glycerol (PPM), is the β'-polymorphic form and there is no β-form. This provided an opportunity to determine the first single crystal structure of TAG β'-polymorph (Sato *et al.*, 2001a). As described earlier in the case of cocoa butter, the functionality of mouth feel and cooling sensation can be interlinked to the physical properties of melting temperature, melting range and enthalpy of melting. These properties emanate from the molecular packing of the high melting β-polymorphic form. In turn the molecular packing and properties can be related to the relative homogeneity in chemical composition and symmetrical TAG structures present as in cocoa butter. The molecular origins of functionality can therefore be understood by relating the chemical structure to the molecular packing and physical properties. The interrelationship of molecular origins of functionality to the properties and chemical structure is shown in Figure 1.8.

Molecular Origins of Functionality

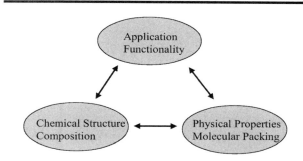

Fig. 1.8. Fundamental knowledge of the influence of chemical structure and composition of a fat on the molecular packing and ensuing physical properties will help to understand the connection between fat functionality and chemical structure.

Studying the molecular structure and packing of groups of compounds where the chemical structure is varied systematically will enhance understanding and could lead to the creation of the ideal fat with desired functionality. There are a number of systematic studies directed to understand the chemical structure to the molecular packing (Fahey *et al.*, 1985; Hagemann *et al.*, 1972; Kodali *et al.*, 1987,1989a, 1990, Sato *et al.*, 2001b; Yano *et al.*, 1999). A few groups of structurally related TAG are presented below.

Molecular Packing and Properties of Monoacid TAG

The physical properties and molecular packing of single acid TAG are listed in Table 1.5. As one would expect, the melting temperatures and enthalpies of these TAG decrease from saturated to monounsaturated to polyunsaturated. Among the monounsaturated the trielaidoyl (*trans*-9) and trivaccinoyl (*trans*-11) gylcerols show considerably higher melting temperatures and enthalpies, making them more suitable for solid fat applications.

The comparison of *cis*, *trans* and saturated monoacid TAG as space-filling models is shown in Figure 1.9. The space-filling models clearly show the packing of saturated TAG, SSS and *trans*-9 TAG, EEE can be facilitated readily compared to the *cis*-9 TAG, OOO with kinked double bonds. All the single acid TAG pack in bilayered structure in the stable β-polymorphic form. However one notable difference between the *trans* unsaturated EEE and saturated, SSS and *cis* unsaturated OOO is that EEE does not form β′-polymorphic form (Kodali *et al.*, 1987). It is possible the *trans* unsaturation may destabilize the orthorhombic subcell packing of β′-polymorphic form. The acyl chain orientation and molecular packing in the layered structure in the stable β-polymorphic form of these TAG will be similar to the published single crystal structure of monoacid TAG, trilauroyl glycerol (Larsson 1964). Typical

TABLE 1.5
The Melting Temperatures and Enthalpies of 18-carbon Single Acid TAG

TAG	Abbreviation[a]	Melting Temp. °C[b]	ΔH of melt[c] Kcal/mole	Packing chain length[d]
Tristearoylglycerol	SSS	73	46	2
Trielaidoylglycerol	EEE	42	36	2
Trivaccinoylglycerol	VVV	42	36	2
Trioleoylglycerol	OOO	5	23	2
Trilinoleoylglycerol	LLL	−13	20	2
Trilinolenoylglycerol	LnLnLn	−24	—	—

[a]S=stearic (C_{18}); E=elaidic ($C_{18:1}$) with *trans* double bond at C9; V=vaccinoyl($C_{18:1}$) with *trans* double bond at carbon 11; O=oleic($C_{18:1}$); L=linoleic ($C_{18:2}$); Ln=Linolenic ($C_{18:3}$).
[b]The melting temperature is of high melting polymorphic form.
[c]The enthalpy of melting is from high melting polymorphic form to melt.
[d]The packing chain length is from powder x-ray diffraction long spacings corresponding to bilayer, two chain length structures (about 45 A).

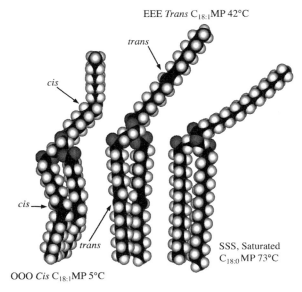

Fig. 1.9. The space-filling models of mono-acid triacylglycerols – tristearoylglycerol (SSS, m.p. 73°C), trielaedoylglycerol (EEE, m.p. 42°C) and trioleoylglycerol (OOO, m.p. 5°C).

representation of layered packing and melting behavior of this class of compounds as represented by SSS and EEE is shown in Figure 1.10.

Molecular Packing and Properties of Symmetric Di-acid TAG

A group of symmetrical di-acid TAG were compared with monoacid TAG, tristearoyl glycerol, SSS and trioleoyl glycerol, OOO. In this group all the fatty acid

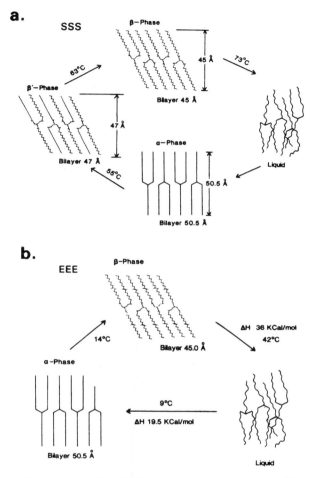

Fig. 1.10. Schematic representation of phase behavior of a. tristearoylglycerol, SSS and b. trielaidoylglycerol, EEE (Kodali *et al.*, 1987).

chains have the same carbon chain length C_{18} but the unsaturation and position of esterification on glycerol differ from each other (Kodali *et al.*, 1987). The nature of the acyl chain at glycerol 2-position influences the melting temperature and enthalpy. The saturated stearoyl chain has a higher melting temparature and enthalpy than the unsaturated chains. Among the unsaturated, the *trans* acid containing TAG have higher enthalpies but the melting temperatures are comparable to *cis* oleic acid containing TAG. The *trans* double bond in the middle of the chain at 9-position in elaidic acid, when moved to 11-position in vaccinic acid, decreases both the enthalpy and melting temperature. This demonstrates that the hydrocarbon chain packing in the methyl end of the chain is more important than the carboxylic acid side. This

TABLE 1.6
The Melting Temperatures and Enthalpies of Di-acid Symmetrical TAG in Comparison to Single Acid TAG, SSS and OOO

TAG	Abbreviation[a]	Melting Temp. °C[b]	ΔH of melt[c] Kcal/mole	Packing chain length[d]
Tristearoylglycerol	SSS	73	46	2
1,3-dioleoyl-2-stearoylglycerol	OSO	25	32	3
1,3-dioleoyl-2-elaidoylglycerol	OEO	9	29	3
1,3-dioleoyl-2-vaccinoylglycerol	OVO	4	23	3
Trioleoylglycerol	OOO	5	23	2

[a]S=stearic (C_{18}); E=elaidic ($C_{18:1}$) with *trans* double bond at C9; V=vaccinoyl ($C_{18:1}$) with *trans* double bond at carbon 11; O=oleic ($C_{18:1}$) with *cis* double bond at C9.
[b]Melting temperature is of high melting polymorphic form.
cThe enthalpy of melting is from most stable β-polymorphic form to melt.
dThe packing chain length is from powder x-ray diffraction long spacings corresponding to bilayer, two chain length structures (about 45 A) or trilayer, three chain length structures (about 65 A).

group also demonstrates that a single *trans* fatty acid chain in a molecule may not be sufficient to increase the enthalpy and melting temperature compared to a *cis* fatty acid chain. The molecular packing of these symmetrical TAG reveal that they pack in trilayered structures. The odd chains at the glycerol 2 position segregate to form a separate layer from the 1 and 3 positions. This acyl chain orientation is similar to monoacid triacyl glycerols even though the latter packs in a bilayered structure. A typical molecular packing of trilayered structure is illustrated by 1,3-dioleoyl-2-stearoylglycerol (OSO) and is shown in Figure 1.11.

Phase Behavior of 1,3-Dioleoyl-2-Stearoylglycerol

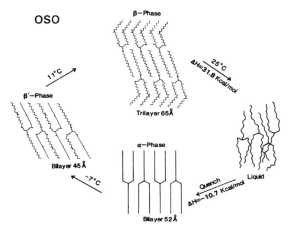

Fig. 1.11. A schematic representation of phase behavior of a di-acid triacylglycerol, OSO (Kodali *et al.*, 1987).

Molecular Packing and Properties of Asymmetric Di-acid TAG

In another systematic study a set of asymmetric di-acid TAG with asymmetric chain substituted at sn-glycerol-3 position were studied (Fahey *et al.*, 1985). The chain length of this 3-acyl chain is increased 2 carbons at a time from C-14, myristic acid, to C-24, lignoceric acid. The physical properties and molecular packing of this series of compounds are compared with trioleoyl glycerol and given in Table 1.7. The melting temperatures and enthalpies of these compounds increase with an increasing chain length. The 3-acyl chain length of C-18 and above show melting temperatures above 20°C but below body temperature. The enthalpies of these compounds are similar to or better than trioleoyl glycerol. The molecular packing of all these compounds reveal trilayered structures with the odd 3-acyl chain segregating from the other two chains to form a middle layer. This trilayer structure packs 1 and 2-acyl chains in the same layer, while the 3-acyl chains of two different molecules form the middle layer. This type of acyl chain packing forces the glycerol conformation perpendicular to the layer plane, which is different from the glycerol conformation of single acid TAG stable crystal structure but similar to diacylglycerols and phospholipids (Goto *et al.*, 1992).

Role of Glycerol Conformation in Molecular Packing and Properties

Understanding the stable glycerol conformation in structurally similar TAG will enable the contribution of glycerol conformation to the stable molecular packing to be understood. The physical properties and packing of OSO and OOS are compared

TABLE 1.7
The Melting Temperatures and Enthalpies of Asymmetric Di-acid TAG in comparison to Single Acid TAG, OOO

TAG	Abbreviation[a]	Melting Temp. °C[b]	ΔH of melt[c] Kcal/mole	Packing chain length[d]
1,2-dioleoyl-3-myristoylglycerol	OOM	12	18	3
1,2-dioleoyl-3-palmitoylglycerol	OOP	18	21	3
1,2-dioleoyl-3-stearoylglycerol	OOS	23	23	3
1,2-dioleoyl-3-arachidoylglycerol	OOA	29	26	3
1,2-dioleoyl-3-behenoylglycerol	OOB	33	28	3
1,2-dioleoyl-3-lignoceroylglycerol	OOLg	36	26	3
Trioleoylglycerol	OOO	5	23	2

[a]M=myristic (C_{14}); P=palmitic (C_{16}); S=stearic (C_{18}); A=arachidic (C_{20}); B=behenic (C_{22}); Lg=lignoceric (C_{24}).
[b]The melting temperature is of high melting polymorphic form.
[c]The enthalpy of melting is from most stable β-polymorphic form to melt.
[d]The packing chain length is from powder x-ray diffraction long spacings corresponding to bilayer, two chain length structures (about 45 A) or trilayer, three chain length structures (about 65 A).

TABLE 1.8

The Melting Temperatures and Enthalpies of Di-acid Symmetric and Asymmetric TAG, OSO and OOS

TAG	Abbreviation[a]	Melting Temp. °C[b]	ΔH of melt[c] Kcal/mole	Packing chain length[d]
1,3-dioleoyl-2-Stearoylglycerol	OSO	25	32	3
1,2-dioleoyl-3-stearoylglycerol	OOS	23	23	3

[a]S=stearic (C_{18}); O=oleic ($C_{18:1}$) with cis double bond at C9.
[b]The melting temperature is of high melting polymorphic form.
[c]The enthalpy of melting is from most stable β-polymorphic form to melt.
[d]The packing chain length is from powder x-ray diffraction long spacings corresponding to trilayer, three chain length structures (about 65 A).

in Table 1.8. The comparison of the molecular packing of symmetric TAG, OSO with asymmetric TAG, OOS shows that both of them pack in trilayered structures. However, to accomplish this, the oleoyl chains segregate from the stearoyl chains to form different layers sandwiching the stearoyl chains, shown in Figure 1.11. This molecular packing forces the glycerol conformation parallel to the layer plane in OSO or perpendicular to the plane in OOS. Except for this difference, the rest of the packing is comparable to each other. The glycerol conformation in these two mole-cules in relation to the end methyl plane is shown in Figure 1.12. This change in

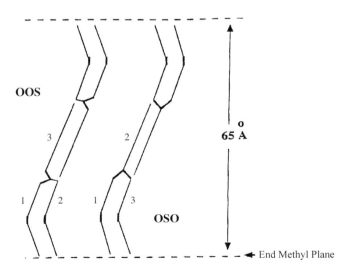

Fig. 1.12. The layered packing of symmetric and asymmetric di-acid TAG OSO and OOS. The 1,2- or 1,3- oleoyl chains of a molecule pack in a layer on either side of stearoyl chains segregated to form a middle layer. This acyl chain arrangement forces the glycerol conformation to be either parallel (OSO) or perpendicular (OOS) to the methyl layer plane.

glycerol conformation influences the enthalpies and melting temperatures of these two compounds. The symmetrical TAG OSO has 2°C higher melting temperature and 9 Kcal/mole higher enthalpy than the asymmetric counterpart.

The glycerol conformation present in OSO is more stable than OOS (Kodali *et al.*, 1987). This is corroborated with the fact that the single crystal structure of monoacid TAG, trilauroylglycerol, shows similar glycerol conformation (Larson 1964). This indicates that when all the three chains are equal, the glycerol conformation parallel to layer plane orientation is preferred. This also confirms the symmetric TAG will have higher melting temperatures and enthalpies than the asymmetric TAG.

Summary

Fats and oils containing TAG are a major class of compounds that are essential not only for various biological functions but also for food functionality. The use of certain oils in the diet is also dictated by the cost and availability. The natural oils and fats contain *cis* double bonds, which isomerise into thermodynamically more stable *trans* form during hydrogenation and deoderization. *Trans* fats, just like saturated fats, offer desirable food functionality. The new FDA regulations stipulate that the *trans* fat content of food products should be included on the label. This created a negative consumer perception of *trans* fats and encourages the food manufacturers to reduce or eliminate the *trans* fats.

There are a number of enabling technologies such as formulation, genetic modification, hydrogenation, fractionation and interesterification that are available to reduce the *trans* fats in food products. However, to create an ideal fat with good food functionality, nutrition, and health, requires an in-depth understanding of structure-properties-functionality relationships. With the existing knowledge in literature fats with one saturated fatty acid / TAG molecule with good functional properties can be produced. To produce ideal fats cost effectively requires leveraging of enabling technologies.

Acknowledgments

The editorial help from Scott Bloomer, Jairajh Mattai and Sithara Kodali is greatly appreciated. I would like to thank the expert assistance of Bassam Jirjis and Gary List in making figures.

References

Ariaansz R.F. and Okonek D.V. *Trans* Isomer Control During Edible Oil Processing. In Proceedings of World Conference on Oilseed Processing, **1.** Ed: S. Koseglu, K. Rhee and R.F. Wilson, AOCS Press, Champaign, IL . 77-91, 1998.

Bailey's Industrial Oil and Fat Products, 5th Edition, Ed: Y.H. Hui, John Wiley and Sons, New York, NY. 1996.

Beers A. and Mangus G. Hydrogenation of Edible Oils for Reduced *Trans* Fatty Acid Content. *Inform.* **15,** 404-405, 2004.

Combe N., Nutritional Implications of *trans* Fatty Acids. 25th World Congress and Exhibition of the International Society of Fat Research (ISF), Abstracts: 2, 2003.

Chapman D. The Polymorphism of Glycerides. *Chem. Rev.* **62**, 433-456, 1962.

Evans C.D., Beal R.E., McConnel D.G., Black L.T. and Cowan J.C. Partial Hydrogenation and Winterization of Soybean Oil. *JAOCS:* **41**, 260-263, 1964.

Fahey D.A., Small D.M., Kodali D.R. Atkinson D. and Redgrave T.G. Structure and polymorphism of 1,2-dioleoyl-3-acyl-*sn*-glycerols. Three- and six-layered structures. *Biochemistry.* **24**, 3757-3764, 1985.

Goto M, Kodali, D.R., Small D.M., Honda K., Kozawa, K., and Uchida, T., Single Crystal Structure of a Mixed-chain Triaclyglycerol: 1,2-Dipalmitoly-3-acetyl-*sn*-glycerol, *Proc. Natl Acad. Sci., USA*, **89**, 8083-8086, 1992.

Gunstone F.D., Harwood J.L. and Padley F.B. The Lipid Handbook. Second Edition, Chapman Hall, 1994.

Hageman J.W., Tallent W.H. and Kolb K.E., Differential Scanning Calorimetry of Single Acid Triglycerides: Effect of Chain Length and Unsaturation. *JAOCS*, **49**, 118-123, 1972.

Hasenhuettl G.L. Fats and Fatty Oils in *Kirk-Othmer Encyclopedia of Chemical Technology*, 4th Edition, Ed., Howe-Grant M. John Wiley & Sons, N.Y. **10**, 252-287, 1994.

Kodali D.R. Vegetable Oil Having Elevated Stearic Acid Content. US Pat. 6,713,117 B1 March 30, 2004.

Kodali D. R. Biobased Lubricants – Chemical Modification of Vegetable Oils. *Inform,* **14**, 121-123, 2003a.

Kodali D.R., Fan Z. and DeBonte L.R. Plants, Seeds, and Oils Having an Elevated Total Monounsaturated Fatty Acid Content. US Pat. 6,649,782 B2 Nov. 18, 2003b.

Kodali D. R., Atkinson D., and Small D. M., Polymorphic Behavior of 1,2-Dipalmitoly-3-lauroyl (PP12)- and 3-myrostoyl (PP14)-*sn*-glycerols, *Journal of Lipid Research*, **31**, 1853-1864, 1990.

Kodali D.R., Atkinson D. and Small D. M. Molecular packing in triacyl-*sn*-glycerols: Influence of acyl chain length and unsaturation. *J. Dispersion Science and Technol.* **10**, 393-440, 1989a.

Kodali D. R., Atkinson D., and Small D. M., Molecular Packing of 1,2-Dipalmitoyl-3-decanoyl-*sn* glycerol (PP10): Bilayer, Trilayer, and Hexalayer Structures, *J. Physical Chemistry*, **93**, 4683-4691, 1989b.

Kodali D. R., Atkinson D., Redgrave T. G., and Small D. M., Structure and Polymorphism of 18-carbon Fatty Acyl Triacylglycerols: Effect of Unsaturation and Substitution in the 2-Position, *Journal of Lipid Research*, **28**, 403-413, 1987.

Kodali D. R., Atkinson D., Redgrave T. G., and Small D. M., Synthesis and Polymorphism of 1,2-Dipalmitoyl-3-acyl-*sn*-glycerols, *JAOCS*, **61**, 1078-1084, 1984.

Larsson K. Solid State Behaviour of Glycerides. *Arkiv For Chemie,* **23**, 35-56, 1964.

List G. R. and King J. W., Hydrogenation in modifying lipids for food use. Ed. F.D. Gunstone, Wood Head Publishing Ltd. UK, in Press, 2005.

Liu K. Soy oil modification: products, applications. *Inform,* **10**, 868-877, 1999.

Loh W. Biotechnology and vegetable oils: First generation products in the marketplace. In Physical Properties of Fats, Oils and Emulsifiers. Ed: N. Widlak. American Oil Chemists Society, AOCS Press, Champaign, IL, 247-253, 2000.

Moss J. S., and Wilkening, V., *Trans* Fat – New FDA regulations. Chapter 2 in *Trans* Fat Alternatives. Ed. Kodali D.R. and List G.R. AOCS Press, Champaign, IL, 26–33, 2005.

Mossoba M.M., Kramer J.K.G., Delmonte P., Yurawecz M. P. and Rader J. I. Official Methods for the Detemination of Trans Fat. AOCS Monograph. AOCS Press, Champaign, IL. 1-22, 2003.

Mounts T.L. Hydrogenation Practices. In Handbook of Soybean Oil Processing and Utilization. Fourth Printing. Ed. Erickson D.R., Pryde E.H., Brekke O.L., Mounts T.M. and Falb R.A. AOCS Press, Champaign, IL. 131-144, 1987.

Pantzaris T. P., Pocketbook of Palm Oil Uses. Fifth Edition. Malaysian Palm Oil Board. Perniagaan Rita, Kaulalampur, 2000.

Redgrave T.G., Kodali D.R. and Small D.M. The effect of triacyl-sn-glycerol structure on the metabolism of chylomicrons and triacylglycerol-rich emulsions in the rat. J. Biol. Chem. 263, 5118-5123, 1988.

Sato K., Goto M., Yano J., Honda K., Kodali D. R. and Small D. M., Atomic Resolution Structure Analysis of Beta Prime Polymorph Crystal of a Triacylglycerol: 1,2-Dipalmitoyl-3-myristoyl-sn-glycerol, Journal of Lipid Research, 42, 338-34 2001a.

Sato K. and Ueno S. Molecular interactions and phase behavior of polymorphic fats, in: Crystallization Processes in Fats and Lipid Systems, ed. N. Garti and K. Sato, Marcel Dekker, New York, pp. 177-209, 2001b.

Sato K. Polymorphism of pure triacylglycerols and natural fats, in: Advances in Applied Lipid Research, vol. 2, ed. F. Padley, JAI Press Inc. New York, pp. 213-268, 1996.

Small D.M. Lateral Chain Packing in Lipids and membranes. Journal of Lipid Research, 25, 1490 – 1500, 1984.

Technical Committee of the Institute of Shortening and Edible Oils, Inc. Food Fats and Oils. Seventh Edition, Institute of Shortening and Edible Oils Inc.,1-29, 1994.

Thomas A. Fats and Fatty Oils. Ullman's Encyclopedia of Industrial Chemistry. 6th Edition, Wiley-VCH, Verlag GmbH & Co. KgaA, Weinheim, 13, 1-73, 2003.

Walter P.K. Working with trans-fat alternatives. Baking Management. March 28-32, 2004.

Yano, Junko., Sato, Kiyotaka., Kaneko, Fumitoshi., Small, Donald M. and Kodali, Dharma R., Structuaral Analysis of Polymorphic Transitions of sn-1,3-Distearoyl-2-Oleoylglycerol (SOS) and sn-1,3-Dioleoyl-2-Stearoylglycerol (OSO): Assessment on Steric Hindrance of Saturated Acyl Chain Interactions. Journal of Lipid Research, 40, 140– 51, 1999.

Chapter 2

Trans Fat—New FDA Regulations

Julie Schrimpf-Moss and Virginia Wilkening

Food and Drug Administration, College Park, MD 20740; julie.moss@fda.gov

This chapter explains the Food and Drug Administration's (FDA or the agency) rule for mandating the labeling of *trans* fatty acids (*trans* fat). This is the first change to the Nutrition Facts panel since the Nutrition Labeling and Education Act of 1990 prompted mandatory nutrition labeling. This chapter also explains the scientific basis that supports the labeling of *trans* fat.

Trans Fat Labeling Proposed Rule

Nutrition Labeling

FDA received a citizen petition in 1994 (Docket No. 1994P-0036/CP1 and LET3) requesting that the agency initiate rulemaking to mandate the addition of *trans* fat to nutrition labeling. The petitioner stated that an increasing body of evidence suggests that dietary *trans* fatty acids raise blood cholesterol levels, thereby increasing the risk of coronary heart disease (CHD). In response to the petition and the growing science associating *trans* fat intake and risk of CHD, FDA issued a proposed rule in 1999 (the 1999 proposal) (DHHS/FDA, 1999). In the 1999 proposal, FDA proposed to amend its nutrition labeling regulation to require, in part, that the amount of *trans* fatty acids in a food or dietary supplement be included when the product contains 0.5 or more grams (g) *trans* fatty acids per serving. Specifically, it proposed the amount of *trans* fat be included in the amount and percent Daily Value (%DV) declared for saturated fatty acids with a footnote indicating the amount of *trans* fatty acids in a serving of the product.

Subsequent to the 1999 proposal, the Institute of Medicine (IOM)/ National Academy of Sciences (NAS) issued a report (IOM/NAS report) (IOM/NAS, 2002) concluding that there is "a positive linear trend" between *trans* fatty acid intake and CHD risk, and recommended that "*trans* fat consumption be as low as possible while consuming a nutritionally adequate diet." The IOM/NAS report did not provide a Dietary Reference Intake (DRI) value for *trans* fat or information sufficient to support the agency establishing a Daily Reference Value (DRV) or other information on the label (i.e., %DV) for *trans* fat. In absence of a basis on which to establish a DV, FDA reopened the comment period of the 1999 proposal (DHHS/FDA, 2002a) to propose to require an asterisk (or other symbol) in the %DV column for *trans* fat, that is tied to a similar symbol at the bottom of the Nutrition Facts box that is followed by the footnote statement "Intake of *trans* fat should be as low as possible." The agency stated that the statement was taken from the IOM/NAS report, was consistent with other recent scientific reports (USDA/DHHS, 2000 and DHHS/NIH, 2002), and was for the purpose of assisting consumers in understanding the quantitative declaration of *trans* fat in the context of a total daily diet.

Nutrient Content and Health Claims

In the 1999 proposal, FDA concluded that dietary *trans* fatty acids have adverse effects on blood cholesterol measures that are predictive of CHD risk (DHHS/FDA, 1999 at p. 62754). Consequently, to avoid misleading claims, the agency proposed that the amount of *trans* fatty acids be limited wherever saturated fat limits are placed on nutrient content claims, health claims, or disclosure and disqualifying levels. FDA also requested comment on whether "*trans* fat free" claims would help consumers maintain healthy dietary practices and whether they would provide incentive to the food industry to reduce the amount of *trans* fat in the food supply (DHHS/FDA, 1999 at p. 62759). FDA proposed a definition for the "*trans* fat free" claim. FDA concluded that there was no basis for defining the claim "low *trans* fat" without a quantitative recommendation for a daily intake of *trans* fat. Further, FDA did not define a "reduced *trans* fat" claim because it was concerned that a reduced *trans* fat claim would detract from educational messages that emphasize lower intakes of saturated fat. However, based on comments received about "reduced *trans* fat" claims, FDA reopened the comment period for the 1999 proposal in December 5, 2000 (DHHS/FDA, 2000) to consider comments that addressed "reduced *trans* fat" and "reduced saturated and *trans* fat" claims.

Scientific Basis

The Dietary Guidelines 2000 (USDA/DHHS, 2000), the National Cholesterol Education Program (NCEP) (DHHS/NIH, 2002) and the IOM/NAS report (IOM/NAS, 2002), based on current scientific evidence, consistently found that *trans* fatty acids are associated with increased LDL-cholesterol levels and that lower intakes of both saturated and *trans* fatty acids are important dietary factors in reducing the risk of CHD in the general population and for those at increased risk for CHD. Thus, there was strong agreement among the expert panels that the available evidence was sufficiently compelling to conclude that *trans* fat intakes increase CHD risk. Accordingly, these expert panels recommended, in addition to their longstanding recommendations that Americans consume diets limited in saturated fat, that consumers also select food products that are low in *trans* fat. These recommendations were made for the general population (Dietary Guidelines 2000 and IOM/NAS report) and persons at increased risk for CHD whose LDL-cholesterol is above goal levels (NCEP). Limiting *trans* fat intake along with saturated fat is also a recommendation from other public health sources, such as the World Health Organization, the American Heart Association and the Dietary Guidelines 2005.

Based on the consistent results across a number of the most persuasive types of study designs (i.e., intervention trials and prospective cohort studies) that were conducted using a range of test conditions and across different geographical regions and populations, the agency concluded that the available evidence for an adverse relationship between *trans* fat intakes and CHD risk was strong (Almendingen *et al.*, 1995; Ascherio *et al.*, 1994; Ascherio *et al.*, 1996; Aro *et al.*, 1995; Aro *et al.*, 1997; de Roos *et al.*, 2001a; de Roos *et al.*, 2001b; Denke *et al.*, 2000; Hu *et al.*, 1997; Judd *et al.*, 1994; Judd *et al.*, 1998; Judd *et al.*, 2002; Kromhout *et al.*, 1995; Lichenstein *et al.*, 1993; Lichenstein *et al.*, 1999; Mensick & Katan, 1990; Nestel *et al.*, 1992; Noakes and Clifton, 1998; Oomen *et al.*, 2001; Pietenin *et al.*, 1997; Roberts *et al.*, 1995; Triosi *et al.*, 1992; Willett *et al.*, 1993; Wood *et al.*, 1993a; Wood *et al.*, 1993b; Zock & Katan, 1992). FDA also found the results from the large prospective cohort studies among free-living U.S. population groups to be persuasive evidence that *trans* fat intakes associated with U.S. dietary patterns can have a significant adverse effect on CHD risk for U.S. consumers. Moreover, independent Federal Government expert panels reviewing the same scientific evidence as FDA consistently concluded that *trans* fat intakes are associated with increased CHD risk and recommend that U.S. consumers and those who need to lower their LDL-cholesterol level minimize their intakes of *trans* fat to reduce their risk of CHD (IOM/NAS report; Dietary Guidelines 2000; NCEP). The scientific agreement for this relationship among the various expert groups provided further evidence of the strength of the science and the public health importance of lowering *trans* fat intakes for U.S. consumers. Therefore, FDA found the overall weight of scientific evidence in support of this conclusion to be sufficiently compelling to warrant *trans* fat labeling so that consumers could know the *trans* fat content of foods and, thereby, make purchase decisions that take dietary recommendations into account.

Trans Fat Final Rule

On July 11, 2003, FDA issued a final rule requiring the mandatory declaration in the nutrition label of the amount of *trans* fat present in foods, including dietary supplements (DHHS/FDA, 2003a). As a result of the many comments to the 1999 proposal strongly opposing the inclusion of *trans* fat as part of the amount and %DV for saturated fat, the agency required that the declaration of *trans* fat be on a separate line immediately under the declaration for saturated fat. It was anticipated that the declaration of this nutrient on a separate line will help consumers understand that *trans* fat is chemically distinct from saturated fat and will assist them in making dietary choices that aid in maintaining healthy dietary practices. The declaration of *trans* fat is to be indented and expressed as grams per serving to the nearest 0.5 gram increment below 5 grams and to the nearest gram increment above 5 grams (see Fig. 2.1). Since there was no scientific basis for establishing a DV for *trans* fat, the final rule did not require the listing of a %DV as is required for some of the other mandatory nutrients, such as saturated fat.

Nutrition Facts
Serving Size 1 cup (228g)
Servings Per Container 2

Amount Per Serving

Calories 260	Calories from Fat 120

	% Daily Value*
Total Fat 13g	**20%**
Saturated Fat 5g	**25%**
Trans Fat 2g	
Cholesterol 30mg	**10%**
Sodium 660mg	**28%**
Total Carbohydrate 31g	**10%**
Dietary Fiber 0g	**0%**
Sugars 5g	

Protein 5g

Vitamin A 4%	•	Vitamin C 2%
Calcium 15%	•	Iron 4%

* Percent Daily Values are based on a 2,000 calorie diet. Your Daily Values may be higher or lower depending on your calorie needs:

	Calories:	2,000	2,500
Total Fat	Less than	65g	80g
Sat Fat	Less than	20g	25g
Cholesterol	Less than	300mg	300mg
Sodium	Less than	2,400mg	2,400mg
Total Carbohydrate		300g	375g
Dietary Fiber		25g	30g

Calories per gram:
Fat 9   •   Carbohydrate 4   •   Protein 4

Fig. 2.1. An example of a Nutrition Facts panel that includes the declaration of *trans* fat.

For the purpose of nutrition labeling, *trans* fats are defined as the sum of all unsaturated fatty acids that contain one or more isolated (i.e., nonconjugated) double bonds in a *trans* configuration. This definition identifies *trans* fatty acids by their chemical structures regardless of origin of the *trans* fatty acid. Under FDA's definition, conjugated linoleic acid would be excluded from the definition of *trans* fat. The definition of *trans* fatty acids, excluding fatty acids with conjugated double bonds, is consistent with the way that *cis* isomers of polyunsaturated fatty acids are defined.

Based on evaluation of more than 1700 comments received, FDA withdrew sections of the 1999 proposal that pertained to the definition of nutrient content claims for "free" and "reduced" levels of *trans* fat and limits on the amounts of *trans* fat wherever saturated fat limits are placed on nutrient content claims, health claims, and disclosure and disqualifying levels. The agency also withdrew the proposed requirement (DHHS/FDA, 2002a) to include a footnote stating: "Intake of *trans* fat should be as low as possible."

The agency set the effective date at January 1, 2006, which is the next uniform effective date following publication of the final rule in 2003 (DHHS/FDA, 2002b). This is the date by which all foods entering interstate commerce must include *trans* fat in the Nutrition Facts panel. This allows firms more than 2 years to implement this final rule, providing some regulatory relief and economic savings for small businesses.

The following are some highlights of the *trans* fat final rule (DHHS/FDA, 2003a at p. 41502-06) that will amend title 21 of the Code of Federal Regulations (CFR) part 101.9 Nutrition Labeling of Food:

- The rule states: "The word "*trans*" may be italicized to indicate its Latin origin." The word "may" is purposely used to allow manufacturers to either italicize the word *trans* or not.
- The rule states: "…except that label declaration of *trans* fat is not required for products that contain less than 0.5 gram of total fat in a serving if no claims are made about fat, fatty acids or cholesterol. … If the serving contains less than 0.5 gram, the content when declared, shall be expressed as zero. …if a statement of the *trans* fat content is not required and, as a result, not declared, the statement "Not a significant source of *trans* fat" shall be placed at the bottom of the table of nutrient values." Therefore, when a product contains zero gram *trans* fat, there are two options. Either label *trans* fat as zero or use the "Not a significant source…" statement. Similarly, the same options apply for saturated fat when a product contains zero gram saturated fat.
- The rule states: "(f) The declaration of nutrition information may be presented in the simplified format set forth herein when a food product contains insignificant amounts of eight or more of the following: Calories, total fat, saturated fat, *trans* fat, cholesterol…." FDA changed the rules regarding the simplified format in 21 CFR 101.9(f) to include *trans* fat in the list of nutrients that may be present at insignificant levels and changed from seven to eight the number that must be insignificant to qualify for the simplified format.
- The rule states: "(5) A food with a label declaration of calories, sugars, total fat, saturated fat, *trans* fat, cholesterol, or sodium shall be deemed to be misbranded under section 403(a) of the act if the nutrient content of the composite is greater than 20 percent in excess of the value for that nutrient declared on the label." FDA changed the rules regarding misbranding in 21 CFR 101.9(g)(5) to include *trans* fat in the list of nutrients that are considered, in part, for compliance with nutrition labeling for food.

Trans Fat Advance Notice of Proposed Rulemaking (ANPR)

Comments received in response to the 1999 proposal were very diverse. Comments relating to claims indicated strongly opposing views. Comments also raised concerns about the absence of consumer studies to determine how the proposed footnote and claims would be perceived. Hence, FDA concluded that based on information and arguments presented in the comments, it was premature to establish new or revised definitions for nutrient content claims or require the use of the proposed footnote statement in the nutrition label. Instead, FDA issued an ANPR on the same day that the *trans* fat final rule was published (Docket No. 2003N-0076) (DHHS/FDA, 2003b) to solicit comment and consumer research on: (1) an appropriate basis for establishing qualifying criteria for *trans* fat in *trans* fat nutrient content claims; current nutrient content claims for saturated fat and cholesterol, lean and extra lean claims; health claims that contain a message about cholesterol-raising lipids; and disclosure and disqualifying levels; (2) whether such claims mislead consumers about the total fatty acid profile if levels of all cholesterol-raising lipids are not addressed, and if qualifiers or disclosure statements would remedy this problem; (3) the use of a footnote or disclosure statement about *trans* fat, either alone or in combination with saturated fat and cholesterol, to enhance consumer understanding; (4) the language that may be appropriate for use in such a footnote or disclosure statement; and (5) the impact of nutrient content or health claims or a footnote or disclosure statement on consumers' food selections.

The agency is currently reviewing comments received as a result of the ANPR (DHHS/FDA, 2003b), conducting consumer research studies and reviewing the current scientific literature. Information obtained will be used by the agency to determine the need for, and content of, further rulemaking on *trans* fat labeling to establish criteria for certain claims (nutrient content or health claims) or to require the use of a footnote, disclosure statement or other labeling approaches about one or more cholesterol-raising lipids in the Nutrition Facts panel to assist consumers in maintaining healthy dietary practices.

References

Almendingen, K., O. Jordal, P. Kierulf, B. Sandstad and J.I. Pedersen. Effects of partially hydrogenated fish oil, partially hydrogenated soybean oil, and butter on serum lipoproteins and Lp(a) in men. *Journal of Lipid Research*, 36:1370–1384, 1995.

Aro, A., A.F.M. Kardinaal, I. Salminen, J.D. Kark, R.A. Riemersma, M. Delgado-Rodriguez, J. Gomez-Aracena, J.K. Huttunen, L. Kohlmeier, B.C. Martin, J.M Martin-Moreno, V.P. Mazaev, J. Ringstad, M. Thamin, P. van't Veer and F.J. Kok. Adipose tissue isomeric *trans* fatty acids and risk of myocardial infarction in nine countries: The EURAMIC study. *Lancet*, 345(8945):273–278, 1995.

Aro, A., M. Jauhiainen, R. Partanen, I. Salminen and M. Mutanen. Stearic acid, *trans* fatty acids, and dairy fat: effects on serum and lipoprotein lipids, apolipoproteins, lipoprotein(a), and lipid transfer proteins in healthy subjects. *American Journal of Clinical Nutrition*, 65:1419–1426, 1997.

Ascherio, A., C. H. Hennekens, J. E. Burling, C. Master, M.J. Stampfer and W.C. Willett. *Trans*-fatty acids intake and risk of myocardial infarction. *Circulation*, 89:94–101, 1994.

Ascherio, A., E.B. Rimm, E.L. Giovannucci, D. Spiegelman, M. Stampfer and W.C. Willett. Dietary fat and risk of coronary heart disease in men: Cohort follow up study in the United States. *British Medical Journal*, 313:84–90, 1996.

de Roos, N.M., M.L. Bots and M.B. Katan. Replacement of dietary saturated fatty acids by *trans* fatty acids lowers serum HDL cholesterol and impairs endothelial function in healthy men and women. *Arteriosclerosis, Thrombosis, and Vascular Biology*, 21: 1233–7, 2001a.

de Roos, N.M., E.G. Schouten and M.B. Katan. Consumption of a solid fat rich in lauric acid results in a more favorable serum lipid profile in healthy men and women than consumption of a solid fat rich in *trans*-fatty acids. *Journal of Nutrition*, 131: 242–245, 2001b.

Denke, M.A., B. Adams-Huet and B.S. Nguyen. Individual cholesterol variation in response to a margarine- or butter-based diet—a study in families. *JAMA*, 284: 2740–2747, 2000.

DHHS/FDA. Food Labeling: *Trans* fatty acids in nutrition labeling, nutrient content claims, and health claims: Proposed Rule. Volume 64 Federal Register, p. 62746, November 17, 1999.

DHHS/FDA. Food Labeling: *Trans* fatty acids in nutrition labeling, nutrient content claims, and health claims: Proposed Rule, reopening of the comment period. Volume 65 Federal Register, p. 75887, December 5, 2000.

DHHS/FDA. Food Labeling: *Trans* fatty acids in nutrition labeling, nutrient content claims, and health claims: Proposed Rule, reopening of the comment period. Volume 67 Federal Register, p. 69171, November 15, 2002a.

DHHS/FDA. Uniform labeling compliance date for food labeling regulations: Final Rule. Volume 67 Federal Register, p. 79851, December 31, 2002b.

DHHS/FDA. Food Labeling: *Trans* fatty acids in nutrition labeling; nutrient content claims, and health claims: Final Rule. Volume 68 Federal Register, p. 41433, July 11, 2003a.

DHHS/FDA. Food Labeling: *Trans* fatty acids in nutrition labeling; consumer research to consider nutrient content and health claims and possible footnote or disclosure statements: Advance Notice of Proposed Rulemaking. Volume 68 Federal Register, p. 41507, July 11, 2003b.

DHHS/NIH. Expert panel on detection, evaluation, and treatment of high blood cholesterol in adults, third report of the National Cholesterol Education Program (NCEP) expert panel on detection, evaluation, and treatment of high blood cholesterol in adults (adult treatment panel III), Chapter II, "Rationale for intervention" and Chapter V "Adopting healthful lifestyle habits to lower LDL cholesterol and reduce CHD risk." 2002 (Internet address: http://www.NHLBI.nih.gov).

Hu, F.B., J. Meir, M.J. Stampfer, J.E. Manson, E. Rimm, G.A. Colditz, B.A. Rosner, C.H. Hennekens and W.C. Willett. Dietary fat intake and the risk of coronary heart disease in women. *New England Journal of Medicine*, 337:1491–1499, 1997.

Institute of Medicine (IOM)/ National Academy of Sciences (NAS). Dietary reference intakes for energy, carbohydrate, fiber, fat, protein and amino acids (Macronutrients). Chapters 8 and 11, National Academy Press, Washington, DC, 2002, p. 335–432 (Internet address: http://www.nap.edu).

Judd, J. T., B.A. Clevidence, R.A. Muesing, J. Wittes, M.E. Sunkin and J.J. Podczasy. Dietary *trans* fatty acids: effects on plasma lipids and lipoproteins of healthy men and women. *American Journal of Clinical Nutrition*, 59:861–868, 1994.

Judd, J. T., D.J. Baer, B.A. Clevidence, R.A. Muesing, S.C. Chen, J.A. Weststrate, G.W. Meijer, J. Wittes, A.H. Lichenstein, M. Vilella-Bach and E.J. Schaefer. Effects of margarine compared with those of butter on blood lipid profiles related to cardiovascular disease risk factors in normolipemic adults fed controlled diets. *American Journal of Clinical Nutrition*, 68:768–777, 1998.

Judd, J.T., D.J. Baer, B.A. Clevidence, P. Kris-Etherton, R.A. Muesing and M. Iwane. Dietary *cis* and *trans* monounsaturated and saturated fatty acids and plasma lipids and lipoproteins in men. *Lipids*, 37:123–131, 2002.

Kromhout, D., A. Menotti, B. Bloemberg, C. Aravanis, H. Blackburn, R. Buzina, A. Dontas, F. Fidanza, S. Giampaoli, A. Jansen, M. Karvonen, M. Katan, A. Nissinen, S. Nedeljkovic, J. Pekkanen, M. Pekkarinen, S. Punsar, L. Räsänen, B. Simic and H. Toshima. Dietary saturated and *trans* fatty acids and cholesterol and 25-year mortality from coronary heart disease: The seven countries study. *Preventive Medicine*, 24:308–315, 1995.

Lichtenstein, A.H., L.M. Ausman, W. Carrasco, J. Jenner, J.M. Ordovas and E.J. Schaefer. Hydrogenation impairs the hypolipidemic effect of corn oil in humans: Hydrogenation, *trans* fatty acids, and plasma lipids. *Arteriosclerosis and Thrombosis*, 13:154–161, 1993.

Lichtenstein, A.H., L.M. Ausman, S.M. Jalbert and E.J. Schaefer. Effects of different forms of dietary hydrogenated fats on serum lipoprotein cholesterol levels. *New England Journal of Medicine*, 340:1933–1940, 1999.

Mensink, R. P. and M. B. Katan. Effect of dietary *trans* fatty acids on high-density and low-density lipoprotein cholesterol levels in healthy subjects. *New England Journal of Medicine*, 323:439–445, 1990.

Nestel, P. J., M. Noakes, G.B. Belling, R. MacArthur, P. Clifton, E. Janus and M. Abbey. Plasma lipoprotein lipid and Lp(a) changes with substitution of elaidic acid for oleic acid in the diet. *Journal of Lipid Research*, 33:1029–1036, 1992.

Noakes, M. and P. M. Clifton. Oil blends containing partially hydrogenated or interesterified fats: differential effects on plasma lipids. *American Journal of Clinical Nutrition*, 68:242–247, 1998.

Oomen, C.M., M.C. Ocke, E.J. Feskens, M-A. van Erp-Baart, F.J. Kok and D. Kromhout. Association between *trans* fatty acid intake and 10-year risk of coronary heart disease in the zutphen elderly study: A prospective population-based study. *Lancet*, 357: 746–51, 2001.

Pietenin, P., A. Ascherio, P. Korhonen, A.M. Hartman, W.C. Willett, D. Algmanes and J. Virtamo. Intake of fatty acids and risk of coronary heart disease in a cohort of Finnish men: The alpha-tocopherol, beta-carotene cancer prevention study. *American Journal of Epidemiology*, 145:876–887, 1997.

Roberts, T.L., D.A. Wood, R.A. Riemersma, P.J. Gallagher and F.C. Lampe. *Trans* isomers of oleic and linoleic acids in adipose tissue and sudden cardiac death. *Lancet*, 345(8945):278–282, 1995.

Troisi, R., W. C. Willett and S. T. Weiss. *Trans* fatty acid intake in relation to serum lipid concentrations in adult men. *American Journal of Clinical Nutrition*, 56:1019–1024, 1992.

U.S. Department of Agriculture (USDA) and DHHS. Nutrition and Your Health: Dietary Guidelines for Americans. 5th ed. Washington DC, Home and Garden Bulletin No. 232, 2000. (Internet address: http://www.health.gov/dietaryguidelines/)

Willett, W.C., M.J. Stampfer, J.E. Manson, G.A. Colditz, F.E. Speizer, B.A. Rosner, L.A. Sampson and C.H. Hennekens. Intake of *trans* fatty acids and risk of coronary heart disease among women. *Lancet*, 341(8845):581–585, 1993.

Wood, R., K. Kubena, B. O'Brien, S. Tseng and G. Martin. Effect of butter, mono- and polyunsaturated fatty acid-enriched butter, *trans* fatty acid margarine, and zero *trans* fatty acid margarine on serum lipids and lipoproteins in healthy men. *Journal of Lipid Research*, 34:1–11, 1993a.

Wood, R., K. Kubena, S. Tseng, G. Martin and R. Crook. Effect of palm oil, margarine, butter, and sunflower oil on the serum lipids and lipoproteins of normocholesterolemic middle-aged men. *Journal of Nutritional Biochemistry*, 4:286–297, 1993b.

Zock, P. L. and M. B. Katan. Hydrogenation alternatives: Effects of *trans* fatty acids and stearic acid versus linoleic acid on serum lipids and lipoproteins in humans. *Journal of Lipid Research*, 33:399–410, 1992.

Chapter 3

Nutritional Considerations of *trans* Fatty Acids[1]

J. Edward Hunter

Department of Chemistry, University of Cincinnati, P.O. Box 210172, Cincinnati, OH 45221-0172; hunterje@email.uc.edu

Introduction

In recent years, *trans* fatty acids (TFA) in foods have received a lot of attention, both in the scientific literature and in the popular press. This attention has come largely from reports that high levels of TFA in the diet, compared to high levels of *cis* fatty acids, have resulted in unfavorable effects on both LDL-cholesterol, the so-called "bad cholesterol," and HDL-cholesterol, the "good cholesterol." In response to these reports, many health professional organizations have recommended reduced consumption of foods containing TFA, and in July 2003, the U.S. Food and Drug Administration (FDA) issued regulations requiring the labeling of TFA on packaged foods on or before January 1, 2006. In addition, many food manufacturers who have used partially hydrogenated oils in their products have developed or are considering ways to reduce or eliminate TFA from these products.

This chapter will cover the following topics: (i) the occurrence of TFA in the U.S. food supply; (ii) three controlled dietary trials relevant to effects of dietary TFA on blood lipid parameters; (iii) a collective look at these and other clinical trials; and (iv) dietary recommendations regarding *trans* and saturated fatty acids by various health professional organizations. The focus will be on TFA in relation to coronary heart disease (CHD) because most of the recent literature on TFA concerns this area of interest.

Figure 3.1 compares structural formulas of the *cis* fatty acid, oleic acid, with its *trans* isomer, elaidic acid. In the *cis* form, the hydrogen atoms are on the same side of the double bond. In the *trans* form they are opposite. As a result of these orientations around the double bond, the *cis* fatty acid has a bend in the carbon chain, whereas the *trans* fatty acid has a straight carbon chain resembling that of a saturated fatty acid.

Occurrence of TFA in the U.S. Food Supply

TFA are formed during partial hydrogenation of fats and oils, a process used to impart desirable stability and physical properties to such food products as margarines

---

[1]The fatty acids of interest in the nutritional studies (e.g., *trans* fatty acids, oleic acid, saturated fatty acids, etc.) were fed as triacylglycerols, not as free fatty acids.

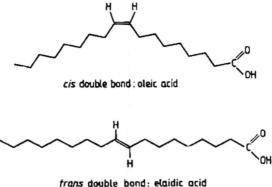

cis double bond: oleic acid

trans double bond: elaidic acid

Fig. 3.1. *Cis* and *trans* fatty acid structural formulas.

and spreads, shortenings, frying fats, and specialty fats (e.g., for fillings, toppings, and candy). In addition, small amounts of TFA occur naturally in foods such as milk, butter, and tallow as a result of biohydrogenation in ruminants.

Typical levels of TFA in food products containing partially hydrogenated oils are shown in Table 3.1. Frying oils used by restaurants and food service operations range in *trans* fatty acid content from zero to about 35% of total fatty acids. Some restaurants and food service operations currently use unhydrogenated oils (such as those used as salad oils) for frying, and such oils are *trans*-free.

Until a few years ago, the fats used in the manufacture of retail margarines and spreads contained, on average, about 15-25% TFA. Currently, most tub, liquid, and spray products contain no *trans* fat. The total fat content of many retail spreads, both tub and stick varieties, currently averages about 55-60%. Thus, these products contain between 0 and 15% TFA by weight. True margarines contain at least 80% fat, but such products now represent only a small market share of the category of margarines and spreads. According to a representative of the National Association of Margarine Manufacturers with whom I spoke, manufacturers of spreads and margarines have reduced *trans* fat levels considerably or eliminated them entirely during the last year or so while holding saturated fat at current levels. This representative

TABLE 3.1
Typical Levels of *trans* Fatty Acids in Food Fats/Products

Food Fat/Product	*Trans* Fatty Acid Content	
Frying fats	0–35% of fatty acids	
Margarines/spreads	fat:	0–25% of fatty acids
	product:	0–15% by wt
Shortenings	0–30% of fatty acids	
Beef and dairy fat	3% of fatty acids	

said that the National Association of Margarine Manufacturers continues to monitor the level of TFA in these products.

Most currently available baking shortenings typically contain about 15-30% TFA, expressed as a percentage of total fatty acids. At least one marketed shortening is *trans*-free. Beef and dairy fat typically contain about 3% TFA, also expressed as a percentage of total fatty acids.

With regard to levels of consumption, Allison *et al.* (1999) reported a mean intake of TFA by the U.S. population of 2.6% of energy, or 5.3 g/person/day. This estimate was based on 24-hour recalls and 2-day food records by over 11,200 subjects as part of the USDA's Continuing Survey of Food Intakes by Individuals. Consistent with these results, Harnack *et al.* (2003) reported that the mean intake of TFA in a population of adult subjects in the Minneapolis-St. Paul, MN, metropolitan area decreased from 3.0% of total energy in 1980-1982 to 2.2% of total energy in 1995-1997. The estimates of Harnack *et al.* were based on 24-hour dietary recalls by more than 7900 subjects participating in the Minnesota Heart Study, an ongoing observational epidemiologic study. These estimated intakes of TFA by Allison *et al.* (1999) and by Harnack *et al.*(2003) of about 2–3% of total energy are small compared to those of saturated fatty acids, which contribute 12–14% of energy intake (Kris-Etherton and Nicolosi, 1995; Anon, 1996; Grundy and Denke, 1990; and Ahuja *et al.*, 1997). The intake of TFA in 14 European countries has been reported to range from 0.5–2.1% of energy, somewhat less than the intake reported for the U.S. (Hulshof *et al.*,1999). This intake of TFA in Europe also is considerably less than the intake of saturated fatty acids in Europe, estimated to be 10–19% of energy (Hulshof *et al.*,1999).

Recent Human Dietary Studies Involving TFA in Relation to Blood Lipoproteins

The following are highlights of three fairly recent controlled human studies which have suggested a relationship between dietary TFA and blood lipoprotein levels. In the first of these studies, Mensink and Katan (1990) had 59 normocholesterolemic subjects (average age 26 years) consume each of three diets for three weeks each. The diets contained typical foods and were similar in nutrient composition except for about 10 percent of total energy, which was provided either as oleic acid, *trans* isomers of oleic acid, or saturated fatty acids (saturates included stearic acid at 3.0–3.6% of energy).

The diet high in TFA resulted in a significant increase in LDL-cholesterol combined with a significant lowering of HDL-cholesterol, compared to the diet high in *cis* fatty acids (the high oleic acid diet). It should be noted, however, that the level of TFA in the high *trans* diet (nearly 11% of energy) was unrealistically high. Nevertheless, the investigators concluded that the effect of TFA on the serum lipoprotein profile was at least as unfavorable as that of cholesterol-raising saturated fatty acids.

Two other carefully controlled studies on effects of dietary TFA on plasma lipid and lipoprotein levels in healthy humans were conducted by Judd and coworkers (1994, 2002). In the first of these studies (Judd *et al.*, 1994), 58 healthy adults (mean age 43 years) consumed each of four diets for six weeks each. One diet contained no TFA (high oleic diet), two contained moderate or high levels of TFA (3.8% or 6.6% of energy, respectively), and the fourth had a high level of saturated fatty acids (16.2% of energy as lauric, myristic, and palmitic acids). The diets were carefully controlled so that the only significant differences between them were the fatty acid compositions of interest.

In this study, both the moderate- and high-*trans* fatty acid diets resulted in increased plasma LDL-cholesterol levels compared to the oleic acid diet. These increases, however, were less than those observed with the saturated fatty acid diet. The high-*trans* diet, but not the moderate-*trans* diet, resulted in a minor (statistically significant) reduction in HDL-cholesterol. The saturated diet, however, led to a slight increase in HDL-cholesterol.

The second study by Judd *et al.* (2002) addressed several limitations of the previous study (Judd *et al.*, 1994). In the second study, a high-carbohydrate diet was included to assess whether direct addition of TFA to the diet had an independent cholesterol-raising effect. Also, a high-stearate diet was included to determine whether stearate and TFA were neutral with regard to their effects on blood lipoproteins. The follow-up study involved 50 healthy male subjects (mean age 42 years), who consumed each of six diets for 5 weeks each. The diets were as follows: high-carbohydrate, high-oleic acid, moderate-*trans* (4% of energy) combined with moderate stearic acid (4% of energy), high-*trans* (8% of energy), high-stearic acid (10.9% of energy), and high-saturated fatty acids (18% of energy as lauric, myristic, and palmitic acids).

Compared to the high-oleic diet, the high-*trans* diet raised LDL-cholesterol to a greater extent (14%) than the high-saturated diet (9%) despite similar levels of *trans* plus saturated fatty acids (18.4% vs. 18.2% of energy, respectively). In contrast, in the previous study (Judd *et al.*, 1994), the increase in LDL-cholesterol after the high-*trans* diet (8%) was directionally (but not significantly) less than that observed after the high-saturated diet (9%); *trans* plus saturates were 16.1% and 16.9% of energy, respectively. Compared to the carbohydrate control diet, both *trans* diets and the saturated diet resulted in increased LDL-cholesterol levels. Considering effects on HDL-cholesterol, the *trans* diets lowered HDL-cholesterol compared to the oleic diet but not compared to the carbohydrate diet. Also compared to the carbohydrate diet, the stearic acid diet had no effect on LDL-cholesterol but lowered HDL-cholesterol. The oleic acid diet had no effect on LDL-cholesterol but raised HDL-cholesterol.

The study by Mensink and Katan (1990) and the two studies by Judd *et al.* (1994, 2002) were consistent in that in all three studies, the *trans* fatty acid and saturated fatty acid treatments raised LDL-cholesterol levels compared to the oleic diet. The changes in LDL-cholesterol levels by TFA and by saturated fatty acids were similar. HDL-cholesterol levels in these studies were reduced consistently when the level of TFA in the diet was 6.6% of energy or higher. In the second study by Judd and colleagues (2002), the moderate *trans* diet showed a reduction in HDL-cholesterol which was not seen in the first study (Judd *et al.*, 1994).

Judd and colleagues noted that while TFA contribute, on average, 2-3% of energy in the U.S. diet (Allison *et al.*, 1999; Harnack *et al.*, 2003), saturated fatty acids contribute 3-4 times more toward the total cholesterol-raising fatty acids in the diet (Grundy and Denke, 1990; Ahuja *et al.*, 1997). Information on the relative importance of saturated fatty acids and TFA with respect to other risk factors, such as clotting tendencies, is needed.

Collective Consideration of Clinical Trials Involving TFA

Other human studies (Zock and Katan, 1992; Nestel *et al.*, 1992; Lichtenstein *et al.*, 1993, 1999; Aro *et al.*, 1997; and Sundram *et al.*, 1997) also have reported increases in LDL-cholesterol levels and decreases in HDL-cholesterol levels when diets high in TFA were compared to diets high in either oleic acid or linoleic acid. Either of these control diets contained only small levels of TFA (from zero to 0.7% of energy).

Nine such studies (Mensink and Katan, 1990; Judd *et al.*, 1994, 2002; Zock and Katan, 1992; Nestel *et al.*, 1992; Lichtenstein *et al.*, 1993, 1999; Aro *et al.*, 1997; and Sundram *et al.*, 1997) have been compared collectively by Ascherio *et al.* (1999). These investigators prepared a graph of the changes in LDL/HDL ratio reported in these studies against the percentage of energy from either TFA or saturated fatty acids (Figure 3.2). Two best-fit regression lines were plotted through the origin, one line representing the percentage of energy from TFA and the other regression line,

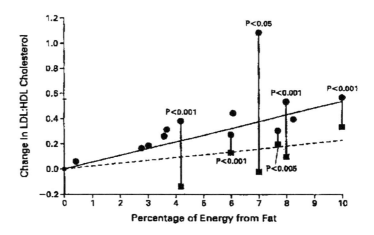

Fig. 3.2. Change in LDL/HDL ratio with level of dietary TFA or SFA. This graph was reported by Ascherio *et al.* (1999) and compares collectively the LDL/HDL ratios against the percentage of energy as either *trans* fat (solid circles, solid line) or saturated fat (solid squares, dashed line) for nine studies (see text).

the percentage of energy from saturated fatty acids. Six of the nine studies (Mensink and Katan, 1990; Judd *et al.,* 1994, 2002; Zock and Katan, 1992; Nestel *et al.,* 1992; Sundram *et al.,* 1997) allowed a comparison between *trans* and saturated fatty acids. Both regression lines had positive slopes, indicating a positive association between intake of either category of fatty acids and CHD risk. However, the slope of the regression line for TFA was larger (by about two-fold) than that for saturated fatty acids. This difference in slopes led the authors to conclude that TFA have a more adverse effect on CHD risk than saturated fatty acids. The conclusion was supported further by the greater effect on LDL/HDL ratio of TFA compared to saturated fatty acids in the six studies that allowed such a comparison. Ascherio *et al.* (1999) suggested that the food industry replace a large proportion of partially hydrogenated fats used in foods and food preparation with unhydrogenated oils.

The studies cited by Ascherio *et al.* (1999) can be considered differently. Figure 3.3 compares the studies based on the levels of TFA and of linoleic acid used in the *trans* fatty acid diet treatments. This scatter diagram indicates that use of relatively high levels of TFA corresponded to use of relatively low levels of linoleic acid. In all cases, the levels of linoleic acid were considered nutritionally adequate, but nevertheless, higher levels of dietary TFA seemed to be associated with lower levels of linoleic acid and vice versa.

Figure 3.4 plots the change in LDL/HDL ratio from the *trans* fatty acid diet treatments cited by Ascherio *et al.* (1999) vs. percentage of energy as linoleic acid. The regression line obtained is opposite in direction (i.e., has a negative slope) compared to the regression line for the percentage of energy as TFA (Figure 3.2). The

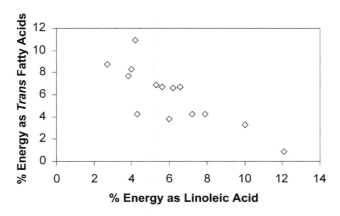

Fig. 3.3. % Energy as TFA and as linoleic acid in TFA diet treatments. This scatter diagram compares the levels of TFA and of linoleic acid used in the TFA diet treatments of the nine studies compared collectively by Ascherio *et al.* (1999). Each open diamond represents the level of dietary TFA and the corresponding level of linoleic acid used in that same treatment.

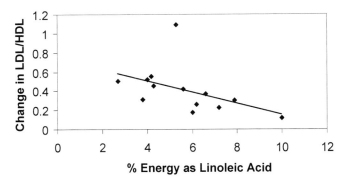

Fig. 3.4. Change in LDL/HDL ratio with level of dietary linoleic acid. This graph plots the change in the ratio of LDL-cholesterol/HDL-cholesterol vs. the dietary level of linoleic acid using data from the nine studies compared collectively by Ascherio *et al.* (1999). The slope for the best-fit regression line is –0.059, similar in magnitude (0.056) to that determined for the graph presented by Ascherio *et al.* (1999) (LDL/HDL ratio vs. % energy as TFA) but opposite in sign.

slope of the best-fit regression line using the linoleic acid data, –0.059 (Figure 3.4), has approximately the same magnitude as the slope of the best-fit regression line using the corresponding *trans* fatty acid data, 0.056 (Figure 3.2).

Several interpretations of the regression line in Figure 3.4 are possible. One interpretation is that the magnitude of the change in LDL/HDL ratio due to TFA may be affected by the level of linoleic acid in the diet. That is, if there is a sufficient level of linoleic acid in the diet, i.e., around 5% to 6% of energy or higher, TFA may be less effective in increasing the LDL/HDL ratio. Another interpretation of Figure 3.4 is that increasing dietary linoleic acid lowers the LDL/HDL ratio through the well-known effect of lowering LDL. However, while the existence of an interaction between linoleic acid and TFA cannot be demonstrated conclusively from the studies cited by Ascherio *et al.* (1999), the possibility of such an interaction cannot be excluded. Additional studies would be needed to clarify this issue.

Forcing the regression line through the origin, as done by Ascherio *et al.* (1999), suggests that Ascherio *et* al believe there is no threshold level of TFA below which there are no unfavorable effects on LDL- or HDL-cholesterol levels. On the other hand, studies with sufficient statistical power to observe small but meaningful population health effects that would establish or exclude a threshold effect of TFA have not yet been published.

Another way to look at these studies collectively is to consider the relationship between simply the change in LDL-cholesterol level or the change in HDL-cholesterol level (rather than the change in their ratio) with increasing level of TFA in the diet. Changes in the LDL/HDL ratio could be due either to changes in LDL-cholesterol or in HDL-cholesterol or in both parameters. Using data from the same nine studies, Figure 3.5 is a scatter diagram I prepared of the change in LDL-cholesterol

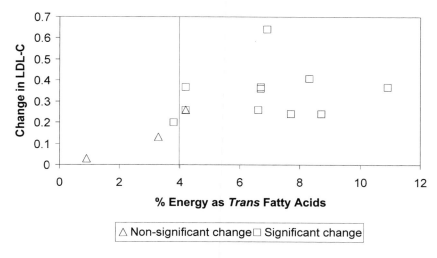

Fig. 3.5. Change in LDL-C with level of dietary TFA. This is a scatter diagram of the change in LDL-cholesterol (expressed as mM) with dietary level of TFA (expressed as % energy) using data from the nine studies compared collectively by Ascherio *et al.* (1999). Changes in LDL-cholesterol were calculated from the difference between a *trans* fatty acid treatment and its corresponding control treatment. Open triangles (△) represent changes in LDL-cholesterol that were reported NOT to be statistically significant. Open squares (□) represent changes in LDL-cholesterol that were reported to be statistically significant.

(in units of mmole/L) with dietary level of TFA. The relationship is directionally similar to that seen when the ratio of LDL/HDL was plotted against the dietary level of TFA (Figure 3.2). Importantly, however, considering these nine studies, the change in LDL-cholesterol was not statistically significant unless the dietary level of TFA was around 4% of energy or higher. Considering the change in HDL-cholesterol (also in units of mmole/L) with increasing level of TFA in the diet (Figure 3.6), with the exception of one study, this change was not statistically significant unless the dietary level of TFA was higher than about 5-6% of energy.

Thus it appears that at a sufficiently high dietary level, TFA indeed raise LDL-cholesterol and reduce HDL-cholesterol levels compared to a diet essentially free of TFA. The dietary levels of TFA necessary to do this appear to be around 4% of energy and higher to increase LDL-cholesterol and around 5-6% of energy or higher to decrease HDL-cholesterol, compared to the control diets.

Dietary Recommendations Regarding Saturated and TFA

Current dietary recommendations by U.S., European, and Japanese health professional organizations address intake of both saturated and TFA. Most of these organi-

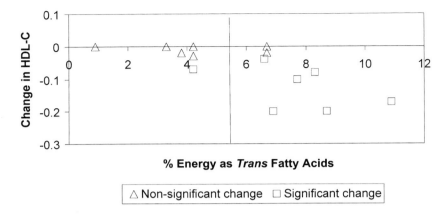

Fig. 3.6. Change in HDL-C with level of dietary TFA. This is a scatter diagram of the change in HDL-cholesterol (expressed as mM) with dietary level of TFA (expressed as % energy) using data from the nine studies compared collectively by Ascherio *et al.* (1999). Changes in HDL-cholesterol were calculated from the difference between a *trans* fatty acid treatment and its corresponding control treatment. Open triangles (△) represent changes in HDL-cholesterol that were reported NOT to be statistically significant. Open squares (□) represent changes in HDL-cholesterol that were reported to be statistically significant.

zations recommend an upper limit of intake of saturated fatty acids of 10% of energy and some recommend an upper limit of intake of TFA of 1-2% of energy.

Recommendations from U.S. organizations are summarized in Table 3.2. The American Heart Association (AHA) suggests (Krauss *et al.*, 2000) that saturated fatty acids make up less than 10% of energy for the population and less than 7% of energy for individuals with elevated LDL-cholesterol or cardiovascular disease. The

TABLE 3.2
Dietary Recommendations: U.S. Organizations

Organization	Saturated Fatty Acids	*trans* Fatty Acids
American Heart Association	<10% en (pop) <7% en (at risk)	Limit so total of cholesterol-raising FA <10% en
Adult Treatment Panel III of the National Cholesterol Education Program	<7% en (at risk)	Keep intake low
Health and Human Services/US Department of Agriculture	<10% en (pop)	Low as possible
Institute of Medicine of the National Academy of Sciences	Low as possible	Low as possible

AHA also recommends limiting intake of TFA from the current level to achieve total intake of cholesterol-raising fatty acids not to exceed 10% of energy. The Adult Treatment Panel III of the National Cholesterol Education Program recently issued a report (Anon, 2001a) applicable to adults with elevated blood cholesterol. This report suggests an intake of saturated fatty acids of less than 7% of energy as part of a therapeutic diet to maximize LDL-cholesterol lowering. It also recommends that intake of TFA be kept low but does not specify an energy limit. The 2005 revision of the U.S. Dietary Guidelines by the Departments of Agriculture and Health and Human Services (Anon, 2005) recommends keeping intake of saturated fatty acids less than 10% of energy and keeping intake of TFA "as low as possible." These organizations also did not specify an energy limit for TFA.

Recently published recommendations from the Institute of Medicine (IOM) of the National Academy of Sciences (Anon, 2002) are consistent with those of other U.S. health professional organizations. The IOM report noted that for *trans* and saturated fatty acids and for cholesterol, there are positive linear trends between intake of each and LDL-cholesterol concentration, and therefore an increased risk of CHD. The IOM report added that TFA, saturated fatty acids, and cholesterol are unavoidable in ordinary diets and that excluding them from the diet would require extraordinary changes in patterns of dietary intake that possibly could introduce undesirable effects. Such dietary adjustments might result in inadequate intakes of certain nutrients and increase certain health risks. Thus for TFA, saturated fatty acids, and cholesterol, the IOM report recommended that intakes be as low as possible from a nutritionally adequate diet.

Among health professional organizations in Europe and Japan (Table 3.3), the Health Council of The Netherlands (Anon, 2001b) has stated that a tolerable upper limit of intake of saturated fatty acids is 10% of energy and that a tolerable upper limit of TFA is 1% of energy. This organization recommends that intakes of both saturated and TFA be kept as low as possible. The UK Ministry of Agriculture similarly

TABLE 3.3

Dietary Recommendations: Non-U.S. Organizations

Organization	Saturated Fatty Acids	*trans* Fatty Acids
Health Council of The Netherlands	Low as possible. UL 10% en[a]	Low as possible. UL 1% en
Health Canada	<10% en	
Ministry of Agriculture, UK	<10% en	<2% en
Austria, Germany, Switzerland	<10% en	
Japan	6-8% en	
World Health Organization/Food and Agricultural Organization of the United Nations	<10% en; <7% en high risk groups	<1% en

[a]en, energy.

recommends an upper limit of intake of saturated fatty acids at less than 10% of energy but a higher upper limit of *trans* fatty acid intake (less than 2% of energy) (Krawczyk, 2001) compared to The Netherlands (less than 1% of energy). Canada, Austria, Germany, Switzerland, and Japan recommend an intake of saturated fatty acids at less than 10% of energy but have not established upper limits of intake of TFA (Krawczyk, 2001).

A report from the World Health Organization and the Food and Agricultural Organization (WHO/FAO) of the United Nations (Anon, 2003) has recommended the traditional target intake of saturated fatty acids (for most people), namely, less than 10% of daily energy intake, and less than 7% for high-risk groups. A very low intake of TFA, less than 1% of daily energy intake, also was recommended. WHO/FAO considers myristic and palmitic acids and TFA to increase the risk of developing CHD.

Because of the agreement among recommendations by many health professional organizations, efforts have been made and are ongoing to decrease TFA in the food supply both in the U.S. and globally.

Summary and Conclusions

In summary, dietary TFA at sufficiently high levels have been found to increase LDL-cholesterol and decrease HDL-cholesterol levels compared to diets high in *cis* monounsaturated or polyunsaturated fatty acids. In general, dietary levels of TFA at around 4% of energy or higher have been found to raise LDL-cholesterol concentrations, and levels of TFA at around 5-6% of energy or higher have been found to lower HDL-cholesterol concentrations. Both of these levels of TFA exceed the reported level of consumption in the U.S. diet of 2.6% of energy. Numerous health professional groups have recommended reduced consumption of TFA. A recent report by the National Academy of Sciences' Institute of Medicine (Anon, 2002) recommends that the consumption of all cholesterol-raising substances, namely, TFA, saturated fatty acids, and cholesterol, be as low as possible in a nutritionally adequate diet.

References

Ahuja, J.K.C., Exler, J., Cahil, P.S., and Raper, N. (1997) *Individual Fatty Acid Intakes: Results from 1995 Continuing Survey of Food Intakes by Individuals*, U.S. Department of Agriculture, Agricultural Research Service, Riverdale, MD.

Allison, D.B., Egan, S.K., Barraj, L.M., Caughman, C., Infante, M., and Heimbach, J.T. (1999) Estimated intakes of *trans* fatty and other fatty acids in the US population, *J. Am. Diet. Assoc. 99*, 166-174.

Anon, ASCN/AIN Task Force on *trans* fatty acids (1996) Position paper on *trans fatty acids*, *Am. J. Clin. Nutr. 63*, 663-670.

Anon, Health Council of the Netherlands (2001b) Dietary reference intakes: energy, proteins, fats and digestible carbohydrates, publication no. 2001/19E, Health Council of the Netherlands, The Hague, pp. 104-109.

Anon, Joint WHO/FAO Expert Consultation on Diet, Nutrition and the Prevention of Chronic Diseases (2003) *Diet, Nutrition and the Prevention of Chronic Diseases*, pp. 87-89, WHO/FAO, Geneva, Switzerland.

Anon, National Cholesterol Education Program (2001a) Third Report of the National Cholesterol Education Program (NCEP) Expert Panel on Detection, Evaluation, and Treatment of High Blood Cholesterol in Adults (Adult Treatment Panel III), NIH publication No. 01-3670, p. V-15, National Heart, Lung, and Blood Institute, National Institutes of Health, Bethesda, MD.

Anon, Panel on Macronutrients, Panel on the Definition of Dietary Fiber, Subcommittee on Upper Reference Levels of Nutrients, Subcommittee on Interpretation and Uses of Dietary Reference Intakes, and the Standing Committee on the Scientific Evaluation of Dietary Reference Intakes, Institute of Medicine of the National Academies (2002) Dietary Fats: Total Fat and Fatty Acids (Chapter 8), in *Dietary Reference Intakes for Energy, Carbohydrate, Fiber, Fat, Fatty Acids, Cholesterol, Protein, and Amino Acids, Part 1*, pp. 8-1–8-97, The National Academies Press, Washington, D.C.

Anon, U.S. Department of Health and Human Services and U.S. Department of Agriculture (2005) Dietary Guidelines for Americans, 2005; 6th edition, Washington, D.C., U.S. Government Printing Office.

Aro, A., Jauhiainen, M., Partanen, R., Salminen, I., and Mutanen, M. (1997) Stearic acid, *trans fatty acids*, and dairy fat: effects on serum and lipoprotein lipids, apolipoproteins, lipoprotein(a), and lipid transfer proteins in healthy subjects, *Am. J. Clin. Nutr. 65*, 1419-1426.

Ascherio, A., Katan, M., Zock, P.L., Stampfer, M.J., and Willett, W.C. (1999) *trans* fatty acids and coronary heart disease, *N. Engl. J. Med. 340*, 1994-1998.

Grundy, S.M., and Denke, M.A. (1990) Dietary influences on serum lipids and lipoproteins, *J. Lipid Res. 31*, 1149-1172.

Harnack, L., Seungmin, L, Schakel, S.F., Duvall, S., Luepker, R.V., and Arnett, D.K. (2003) Trends in the *trans*-fatty acid composition of the diet in a metropolitan area: The Minnesota Heart Study, *J. Am. Diet. Assoc. 103*, 1160-1166.

Hulshof, K.F.A.M., van Erp-Baart, M.A., Anttolainen, M., Becker, W., Church, S.M., Couet, C., Hermann-Kunz, E., Kesteloot, H., Leth, T., Martins, I., Moreiras, O., Moschandreas, J., Pizzoferrato, L., Rimestad, A.H., Thorgeirsdottir, H., van Amelsvoort, J.M.M., Aro, A., Kafatos, A.G., Lanzmann-Petithory, D., and van Poppel, G. (1999) Intake of fatty acids in Western Europe with emphasis on *trans fatty acids*: the TRANSFAIR study, *Eur. J. Clin. Nutr. 53*, 143-157.

Judd, J.T., Baer, D.J., Clevidence, B.A., Kris-Etherton, P., Muesing, R.A., and Iwane, M. (2002) Dietary *cis* and *trans* monounsaturated and saturated fatty acids and plasma lipids and lipoproteins in men, *Lipids 37*, 123-131.

Judd, J.T., Clevidence, B.A., Muesing, R.A., Wittes, J., Sunkin, M.E., and Podczasy, J.J. (1994) Dietary *trans fatty acids*: effects on plasma lipids and lipoproteins of healthy men and women, *Am. J. Clin. Nutr. 59*, 861-868.

Krauss, R.M., Eckel, R.H., Howard, B., Appel, L.J., Daniels, S.R., Deckelbaum, R.J., Erdman, J.W., Kris-Etherton, P., Goldberg, I.J., Kotchen, T.A., Lichtenstein, A.H., Mitch, W.E., Mullis, R., Robinson, K., Wylie-Rosett, J., St. Jeor, S., Suttie, J., Tribble, D.L., and Bazzarre, T.L. (2000) AHA Dietary Guidelines. Revision 2000: A statement for health-care professionals from the Nutrition Committee of the American Heart Association, *Circulation 102*, 2296-2311.

Krawczyk, T. (2001) Fat in dietary guidelines around the world, *Inform 12*, 132-140.

Kris-Etherton, P.M., and Nicolosi, R.J. (1995) *trans Fatty Acids and Coronary Heart Disease Risk*, pp. 1-24, International Life Sciences Institute, Washington, D.C.

Lichtenstein, A.H., Ausman, L.M., Carrasco, W., Jenner, J.L., Ordovas, J.M., and Schaefer, E.J. (1993) Hydrogenation impairs the hypolipidemic effect of corn oil in humans. Hydrogenation, *trans* Fatty Acids, and plasma lipids, *Arteriosclerosis and Thrombosis 13*, 154-161.

Lichtenstein, A.H., Ausman, L.M., Jalbert, S.M., and Schaefer, E.J. (1999) Effects of different forms of dietary hydrogenated fats on serum lipoprotein cholesterol levels, *N. Engl. J. Med. 340*, 1933-1940.

Mensink, R.P., and Katan, M.B. (1990) Effects of dietary *trans* fatty acids on high-density and low-density lipoprotein cholesterol levels in healthy subjects, *N. Engl. J. Med. 323*, 439-445.

Nestel, P., Noakes, M., Belling, B., McArthur R., Clifton, P., Janus, E., and Abbey, M. (1992) Plasma lipoprotein lipid and Lp[a] changes with substitution of elaidic acid for oleic acid in the diet, *J. Lipid Res. 33*, 1029-1036.

Sundram, K., Ismail, A., Hayes, K.C., Jeyamalar, R., and Pathmanathan, R. (1997) *Trans* (elaidic) fatty acids adversely affect the lipoprotein profile relative to specific saturated fatty acids in humans, *J.Nutr. 127*, 514S-520S.

Zock, P.L., and Katan, M.B. (1992) Hydrogenation alternatives: effects of *trans* fatty acids and stearic acid versus linoleic acid on serum lipids and lipoproteins in humans, *J. Lipid Res. 33*, 399-410.

Chapter 4

Determination of *trans* Fats by Gas Chromatography and Infrared Methods

Magdi Mossoba, John K.G. Kramer, Pierluigi Delmonte, Martin P. Yurawecz, and Jeanne I. Rader

United States Food and Drug Administration, College Park, MD 20742;
Magdi.Mossoba@fda.hhs.gov

Introduction

Labeling of the *trans* fatty acid content of foods is currently being considered in many countries. Labeling of *trans* fat became mandatory in Canada in January 2003 (http://canadagazette.gc.ca/partII/2003). The U.S. Food and Drug Administration will soon issue a final rule on the labeling of the *trans* fatty acid content of food products. A voluntary reduction of total *trans* fats in food products was introduced in the European Union in the late 1990s, while Australia and New Zealand are currently considering this issue.

In this chapter, the latest approved gas chromatographic and infrared spectroscopic official methods used to determine *trans* fatty acids will be reviewed. In addition, a brief discussion is included about analytical procedures that have also been applied to the quantitation of *trans* fatty acids in food products. Further studies are still needed to address outstanding issues, namely differences in the total *trans* fatty acid content obtained by gas chromatographic and infrared spectroscopic techniques, the applicability of methods to determine the *trans* content in different food matrices, and the development of methods to analyze *trans* isomers with potentially beneficial physiological effects.

Structure and Occurrence of *trans* Fatty Acids

Trans fatty acids are carboxylic acids with a long hydrocarbon chain in which the isolated double bond occurs in the *trans* configuration (Fig. 4.1). The position of the double bond is defined relative to C1, the carboxyl group carbon atom. For example, elaidic acid (*trans* 9-18:1) is a C18 fatty acid in which the *trans* double bond occurs between C9 and C10. Positional isomers are C18 fatty acid structures in which the unsaturated sites occur between different pairs of adjacent carbon atoms along the hydrocarbon chain. All of the unsaturated sites in natural fats and oils from plant or animal origins generally occur in the *cis* double bond configuration, such as oleic acid (*cis* 9-18:1), in which a *cis* double bond occurs between C9 and C10 of the C18 fatty acid hydrocarbon chain.

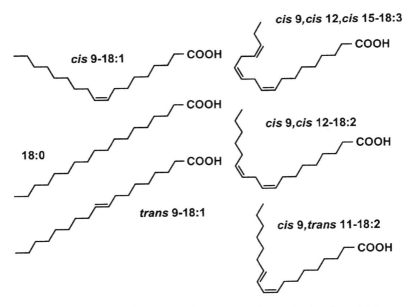

Fig. 4.1. Chemical structures for common fatty acids in oils and fats.

Trans fat is found naturally in ruminant fat as a result of polyunsaturated fatty acids (PUFA) isomerization by rumen bacteria in ruminants. They range in level from 1 to 8% (as percent of total fat) in dairy products and red meats from beef and sheep (Wolff *et al.*, 1998; Craig-Schmidt, 1998). The other major source of *trans* fatty acids occurs during partial hydrogenation of vegetable oils (Craig-Schmidt, 1998). Levels of *trans* fat of up to 50% (as percent of total fat) have been reported in products containing partially hydrogenated vegetable oils (PHVO) (Table 4.1) (Fritsche and Steinhart, 1997). During the deodorization step in the refinement of vegetable oils, *trans* levels of approximately 3% (as percent of total fat) are generally produced originating from isomerization of linoleic *cis* 9,*cis* 12-18:2) and linolenic (*cis* 9,*cis* 12,*cis* 15-18:3) acids into *trans* geometric isomers (Fritsche and Steinhart, 1997). *Trans* 18:1 isomers represent over 80% and 90% of total *trans* fats in ruminant fats and partially hydrogenated vegetable oils, respectively (Wolff and Precht, 2002).

Fats from various sources differ not only in the amount of *trans*-18:1 fat, but more importantly in the relative distribution (Wolffe, 1998; Fritsche 1997) of the different positional isomers (Figs. 4.2–4.4). While PHVO show a more even distribution of the *trans*-18:1 isomers from *trans* 6-8 to *trans* 13-14-18:1 (Fig. 4.2), the distribution of *trans*-18:1 isomers in dairy fats shows *trans* 11-18:1 as the major *trans*-18:1 isomer (Fig. 4.3) (Chardigny *et al.*, 1996; Precht and Molkentin, 1999). The distribution of *trans*-18:1 isomers in human milk may reflect the relative intake of dairy fats or PHVO in the diet of the mother (Wolff, 1995). Figure 4.4 shows a profile of human milk fat that resembles that of PHVO.

TABLE 4.1
Ranges of *trans* Fat Contents for Selected Food Products

Product	*Trans* 18:1 (% total fat)	Total *trans* (% total fat)
Stick margarine, soy	19–41	19–49
Tub margarine, soy	9–21	11–28
Shortening, soy	9–27	3–30
Cooking oil, soy	5–11	1–13
Salad oil, soy	0–3	0–5
Cookies	3–32	4–36
Cake	9–11	10–13
Milk shake	2–3	2–4
Hamburger	3–5	3–5
Potato chips	0–34	0–40
French fries	3–32	3–34
Butter	2–6	2–7
Whole milk	2–3	2–4
Beef	2–5	2–5

Dairy fats are the major source of conjugated linoleic acids (CLA) which contain one *trans* and one *cis* double bond separated by a single bond, such as *cis* 9,*trans* 11-18:2 (Fig. 4.1), and *trans* 7,*cis* 9-18:2 (Yurawecz *et al.*, 1998). The content of CLA in ruminant fat can range from 0.5 to 2% (as percent of total fat) depending on

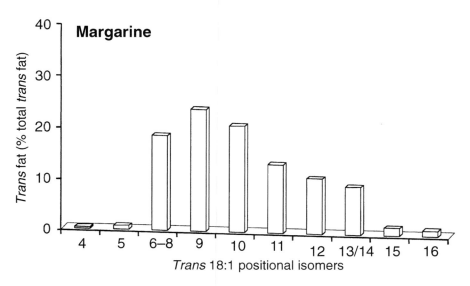

Fig. 4.2. Relative distribution of *trans* 18:1 positional isomers in margarine.

M.M. Mossoba et al.

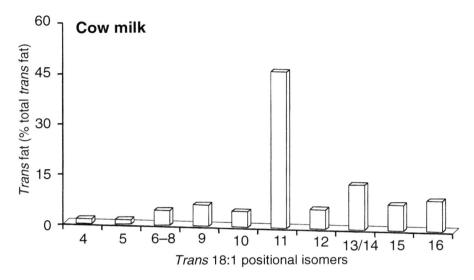

Fig. 4.3. Relative distribution of *trans* 18:1 positional isomers in cow milk.

the diet fed to animals (Wolff, 1995; Precht and Molkentin, 2000). CLA isomers have been reported to have anticarcinogenic properties and other beneficial physiological effects in animal studies (Pariza *et al.*, 2001).

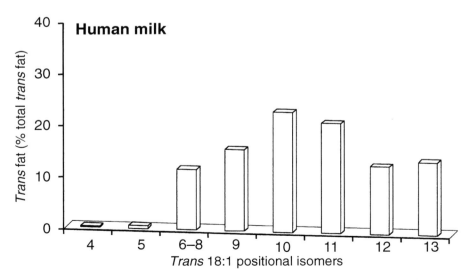

Fig. 4.4. Relative distribution of *trans* 18:1 positional isomers in human milk.

Official Methods

Capillary Gas Chromatography

Gas chromatography (GC) has been the most widely used analytical method to analyze fatty acid methyl esters (FAME) (Wolff and Precht, 2002; Chardigny *et al.*,
1996; Precht and Molkentin, 1999; Wolff, 1995; Henninger and Ulberth, 1994;
Duchateau, 1996; Ratnayake, 2001; Kramer *et al.*, 2002). A successful GC determination of total *trans* FAME composition depends on the experimental conditions dic-
tatedby the method used, as well as sound judgment by the analyst to identify peaks
attributed to *trans* FAME and their positional isomers correctly. The most recent GC
methods to determine *trans* FAME describe separations that require long capillary
columns with highly polar stationary phases. Under these conditions, a separation is
based on the chain length of the fatty acid, degree of unsaturation, and the geometry
and position of double bonds. The expected elution sequence for specific fatty acids
with the same chain length on highly polar columns is as follows: saturated, monounsaturated, diunsaturated, etc. *Trans* positional isomers are followed by *cis* positional
isomers, but there is extensive overlap of the geometric isomers.

The improved resolution of the large number of peaks attributed to *trans* and *cis*
positional isomers obtained under today's optimal experimental conditions, leads to
the partial or complete overlap of many peaks belonging to the two different groups
of geometric isomers) (Wolff and Precht, 2002; Precht and Molkentin, 1999; Wolff,
1995; Henninger and Ulberth, 1994; Duchateau, 1996; Ratnayake, 2001; Kramer *et
al.*, 2002). This is because the retention time range for late eluting *trans* 18:1 positional isomers, starting at $\Delta12$ (or $\Delta13$ depending on experimental conditions used),
is the same as that for the *cis* 18:1 positional isomers, $\Delta6$–$\Delta14$. In addition, *cis/trans*
18:2 methylene- and non-methylene interrupted fatty acid retention time range over-
laps with that of the *cis*-18:1 positional isomers. Typical FAME profiles with over-
lapping *trans*-18:1, *cis*-18:1 and *cis/trans* 18:2 isomers for total milk fat and PHVO
are shown in Figures 5 and 6, respectively.

Elimination of GC peak overlap usually requires prior separation of the *cis* and
trans 18:1 geometric isomers by silver ion-TLC (Wolff and Precht, 2002; Chardigny *et
al.*, 1996; Precht and Molkentin, 1999; Wolf, 1995; Henninger and Ulberth, 1994;
Kramer *et al.*, 2002; Kramer *et al.*, 2001; Buchgraber and Ulberth, 2001). GC analysis
of the isolated *trans* and *cis* fractions indicates the extent of overlap (Fig. 4.7). Most
individual 18:1 isomers can be completely resolved by GC under isothermal conditions
at much lower temperatures (Fig. 4.8) (Wolff and Precht, 2002; Precht and Molkentin,
1999; Kramer *et al.*, 2002; Kramer *et al.*, 2001; Buchgraber and Ulberth, 2001).

The effect of this GC peak overlap on the accuracy of *trans* FAME determinations for ruminant fats and PHVO depends on (a) the nature of the *trans* fat being
analyzed, because the isomeric distributions of natural fats (such as milk fat) and
PHVO are determined by the nature of the source fat or oil and/or hydrogenation and
processing conditions; (b) the GC experimental conditions (nature, length, and age of

column, carrier gas, temperature program, etc.); and (c) the analyst's experience and skill in optimizing and evaluating the performance of the gas chromatographic system, and subsequently identifying all the observed GC peaks in widely different and complex chromatographic profiles, after calibration with as many reference standards as available commercially or otherwise.

GC Official Methods AOAC 996.06 and AOCS Ce 1f-96. GC methods determine fatty acids as percent of total fatty acids, whereas a more quantitative analysis is needed for food labeling purposes. Thus, an internal standard must be added to the food matrix prior to GC analysis. GC official method AOAC 996.06 (AOAC International, 1997) is appropriate for the determination of fat in food products, while AOCS Ce 1f-96 (AOCS, 1999) is applicable to the determination of *cis* and *trans* fatty acids in hydrogenated and refined vegetable oils and fats.

Briefly, official method AOAC 996.06 (AOAC International, 1997) describes procedures to extract fat and fatty acids from foods by hydrolytic methods. These include acidic hydrolysis for most foods, alkaline hydrolysis for dairy products, and a combination of these procedures for cheese. To minimize oxidative degradation of fatty acids during analysis, AOAC method 996.06 requires the addition of pyrogallic acid. Triundecanoin (11:0), diethyl ether, and boron trifluoride are used as internal standard, for extraction of fat and methylation, respectively. AOAC method 996.06 states that the highly polar stationary phase SP-2560 (100 m . 0.25 mm id, 0.20 μm film) column from Supelco Inc. (Bellefonte, PA, USA) is suitable for this determination. Total fat is obtained from the sum of all individual fatty acids (including *trans*-monoenes) expressed as triglyceride equivalent. Saturated and only *cis*-monounsaturated fats are calculated from the sum of their respective components. Identification is based on comparison with commercial standards; these must all be purchased from the same supplier. Unknown components should not be included in the summation, unless they can first be identified by mass spectrometry and/or infrared spectroscopy. It would be possible for an analyst to extend this methodology and calculate *trans*-monounsaturates from the sum of their respective components, as detailed in the latest official method AOCS Ce 1f-96 (AOCS, 1999).

Using a single capillary GC analysis, AOCS Ce 1f-96 (AOCS, 1999) provides qualitative and quantitative determinations for *trans* fatty acid isomers, as well as saturated fatty acids (SAFA), monounsaturated fatty acids (MUFA), and polyunsaturated fatty acids (PUFA). AOCS method Ce 1f-96 (AOCS, 1999) states that either a short (50 or 60 m) or a long (100 or 120 m) column with a highly polar stationary phase may be used, for example, CP-Sil 88, 100 or 50 m . 0.25 mm id, 0.20 μm film (Fig. 4.9) from Chrompack, (Middleburg, the Netherlands), SP-2560, 100 or 50 m . 0.25 mm id, 0.20 μm film from Supelco Inc. (Bellefonte, PA, USA), or BPX-70, 120 or 50 m × 0.22 mm id, 0.25 μm film from SGE, Inc. (Austin, TX, USA). AOCS method Ce 1f-96 also requires a gas chromatograph equipped with a capillary injector that can provide a split ratio of approximately 1:100 and a flame ionization detector (FID), both operating at 250°C.

The isothermal oven temperature, column head pressure, and the carrier gas (He) linear velocity depend on the column used, for example, 170°C, 125 kPA, 16 cm/sec for SP-2560, 175°C, 130 kPa, 19 cm/sec for CP-Sil 88, and 19°C, 155 kPa, 17 cm/sec for BPX-70. The carrier gas may be helium, nitrogen, or hydrogen. The boron trifluoride method (AOCS Ce 2-66 or IUPAC 2.301) should be used to prepare FAME from triacylglycerols of fats and oils. The specified internal standard is 5 mg tridecanoin/mL chloroform.

AOCS method Ce 1f-96 also states that system optimization may be required first. Small corrections may be needed if the observed chromatogram for a test sample does not match the published profile of a typical standard mixture obtained under the method's optimal conditions. According to AOCS method Ce 1f-96, this refinement would correct batch differences between column performance and instrument temperature control. Specifically, for a 0.5–1.0 µL injection of a 7 mg/mL test sample, a 1°C stepwise increase or decrease in oven temperature is recommended until a match is found between the chromatographic traces. For example, with most of the columns specified by the method, a slight increase in temperature would further resolve the adjacent pair of peaks attributed to *cis*-20:1 and *cis,cis,cis*-18:3 by leading to a shorter retention time of the first peak relative to the second (Fig. 4.10).

Once optimized, the performance of the system should be evaluated according to AOCS method Ce 1f-96 (AOCS, 1999). For partially hydrogenated fats and oils (Figs. 4.6 and 4.9), the recommended test consists of checking whether the very weak peak due to the coeluting Δ13 and Δ14-*trans* FAME positional isomers is partially resolved from that of the intense Δ9 *cis*-18:1 FAME positional isomer (Figs. 4.5 and 4.6). For oils refined at high temperatures (Fig. 4.10), the analyst should observe whether (a) the intense Δ9 *cis*-18:1 and the adjacent but much weaker Δ11 *cis*-18:1 FAME positional isomeric peaks are clearly separated; (b) the peak due to 20:1 is positioned exactly between those of the last eluting methyl linolenate geometric isomer, *trans,cis,cis*-18:3, and *cis,cis,cis*-18:3; and (c) seven relatively weak *trans* peaks are observed due to the isomers Δ9 *trans*-18:1; Δ9,Δ12 *cis,trans*- and, *trans,cis*-18:2; and Δ9,Δ12,Δ15-*trans,cis,trans*-, *cis,cis,trans*-, *cis,trans,cis*-, and *trans,cis,cis*-18:3 FAME (Figs. 4.10 and 4.11). These seven peaks should also be used to identify the *trans* components of refined oils. For the more complex profiles of partially hydrogenated oils, the equivalent chain length (ECL) rules should be applied for identification, after appropriate calibration with *cis* and *trans* standards of FAME and their positional isomers.

Quantitative GC Determination of trans *Fatty Acids.* Once identified, the quantitative determination of all *trans* GC components is carried out as follows (AOCS, 1999) . Each peak area is corrected to compensate for the FID response. For each FAME component (x), the FIDx correction factor is calculated from its molecular weight (MWx), (nx^{-1}), where (nx) is the number of carbon atoms, the atomic weight of carbon (AWc), 12.01, and the 16:0 correction factor (FID16:0), 1.407, according to the relation:

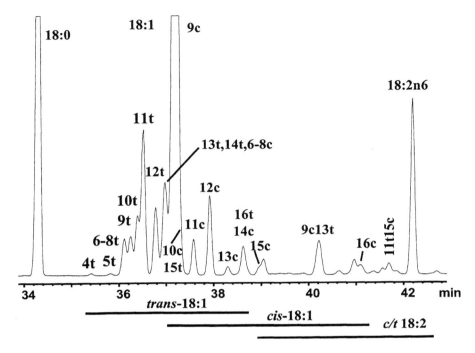

Fig. 4.5. Partial GC FAME profile (18:0 to 18:2) for total milkfat using a 100-m CP-Sil 88 column and a temperature program from 45 to 215°C (Kramer 2001, 2002). The partial overlap of *trans*-18:1, *cis*-18:1, and *cis/trans* 18:2 isomers is indicated.

$$FIDx = MWx/(nx^{-1}) \, (AWc) \, (FID16:0)$$

A corrected area (Ax) is obtained by multiplying a given peak area by its correction factor. The amount (Xx) of a FAME component is determined (as percent of total FAME) as follows:

$$Xx = Ax/At$$

where (At) is the sum of all corrected peak areas, excluding the solvent peak, and the total *trans* level is calculated as the sum of all the *trans* components in a given mixture.

Prefractionation of Trans *18:1 Geometric Isomers by Silver Ion Chromatography.* The separation and quantitation of total *trans* fatty acids in ruminant fats (Fig. 4.5), human milk, and partially hydrogenated fats and oils (Fig. 4.6), by GC as FAME using long highly polar capillary columns considerably underestimates the C18 *trans*-mononounsaturated FAME (*trans*-18:1) content by the amount of Δ12- to Δ16-18:1 *trans*

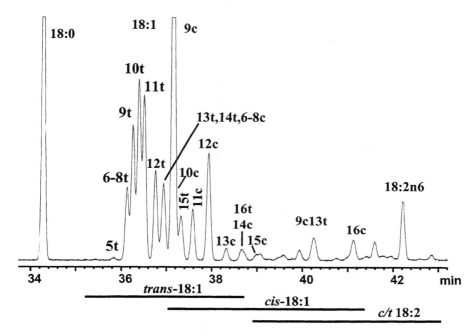

Fig. 4.6. Partial GC FAME profile (18:0 to 18:2) for a partial hydrogenated vegetable oil using a 100-m CP-Sil 88 column and a temperature program from 45 to 215°C (Kramer *et al.*, 2002; Kramer *et al.*, 2001). The partial overlap of *trans*-18:1, *cis*-18:1, and *cis/trans* 18:2 isomers is indicated.

FAME positional isomers (Wolff and Precht, 2002; Precht and Molkentin, 1999; Kramer *et al.*, 2002; Kramer *et al.*, 2001). This is because several of these *trans* isomers partially or completely overlap with *cis*-18:1 positional isomers (Fig. 4.7).

Silver ion-thin layer chromatography (Ag⁺-TLC) (Wolff and Precht, 2002; Chardigny *et al.* 1996; Precht and Molkentin, 1999; Wolff, 1995; Henninger and Ulberth, 1994; Kramer *et al.*, 2002; Kramer *et al.*, 2001) or Ag⁺-high pressure liquid chromatography (Ag⁺-HPLC) (AOCS official method Ce 1g-96) (AOCS, 1999a) can be used to overcome this overlap problem by completely fractionating the *trans* from the *cis*-18:1 geometric isomers (Figs. 4.7 and 4.8) prior to the GC determination (Wolff and Precht, 2002; Precht and Molkentin, 1999; Kramer *et al.*, 2002; Kramer *et al.*, 2001; Buchgraber and Ulberth, 2001). The adverse impact on accuracy due to the GC peak overlap can also be overcome by applying infrared spectroscopy to determine the *trans* fats.

Fourier-Transform Infrared Spectroscopy

Instrumentation. A brief introduction of today's infrared technology will help the reader understand the *trans* fat methodologies reviewed below. A Fourier transform

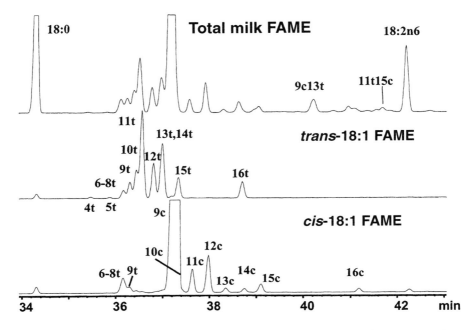

Fig. 4.7. Partial GC FAME profile (18:0 to 18:2) for total milkfat, and the *trans* and *cis* fractions isolated by silver ion-TLC. A 100-m CP-Sil 88 column was used, and a temperature program from 45 to 215°C (Kramer *et al.*, 2001, 2002). Note the presence of the Δ6-9 *trans* 18:1 positional isomers in the *cis* fraction.

infrared (FTIR) spectrometer (Reedy and Mossoba, 1999) consists of a source of continuous infrared radiation that emits light from a high temperature element that withstands prolonged heating and exposure to air, an interferometer, and a detector. The interferometer allows the detection of all the component wavelengths of the mid-infrared region (4000–600 cm^{-1}) simultaneously. When a test sample (such as a *trans* fat solution) is placed between the beam splitter and the detector, it selectively absorbs infrared energy. Changes in the energy reaching the detector as a function of time yield an interferogram, the raw infrared spectrum. When the interferogram is converted from the time to the frequency domain by the mathematical Fourier transformation, a single-beam spectrum (Fig. 4.12) is obtained. The single-beam spectrum of a "test sample" is the emittance profile of the infrared source as well as the absorption bands of all infrared-absorbing material in the path of the infrared beam, namely the test sample, atmospheric water vapor, and CO_2. A "background" (such as a solvent or a *trans*-free fat solution) single-beam spectrum is also measured. To observe the conventional transmission (or absorption) spectrum of a test sample (Fig. 4.13), the single-beam spectrum of the test sample is digitally "ratioed" against the single-beam spectrum of the reference background.

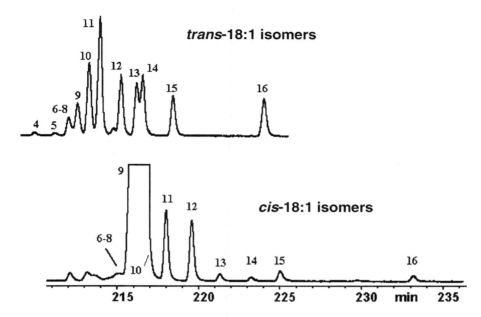

Fig. 4.8. *Trans* and *cis* 18:1 positional isomers GC FAME profiles for butter using a 100-m CP-Sil 88 column recorded under conditions that are optimal for the resolution of the Δ13 and 14 *trans* 18:1 positional isomers (Kramer *et al.*, 2002; Kramer *et al.*, 2001). The *trans* and *cis* fractions were first separated by silver ion-TLC.

FTIR instrumentation offers several advantages over dispersive spectrometers that use prisms or diffraction gratings to resolve the infrared light into its component wavelengths (Reedy and Mossoba 1999). An entire FTIR spectrum can be measured in a single scan in about 1 sec. A high signal-to-noise ratio can be typically achieved in 1–2 min. Wavelength precision is provided by an internal reference laser. The computing capabilities offer powerful data-handling and quantitative manipulation routines. The higher energy throughput allows the efficient use of different sample handling techniques, such as attenuated total reflection (ATR) (Harrick, 1967; Internal Reflection Spectroscopy, 1992; Ismail *et al.*, 1998).

Transmission Mode. In the standard transmission mode (Reedy and Mossoba, 1999; Ismail *et al.*, 1998), certain frequencies are absorbed as the infrared beam passes through the test sample, and only the transmitted light reaches the detector and is measured. Transmission liquid cells have traditionally been used to determine *trans* fats. They are made of a pair of salt crystals (such as NaCl) that are separated by a thin Teflon spacer. As indicated by Beer's law, $A = a \cdot b \cdot c$, the absorbance (A) depends on the molar absorption coefficient at a particular wavelength (a), the pathlength of infrared light through the test sample (b) that is dictat-

M.M. Mossoba et al.

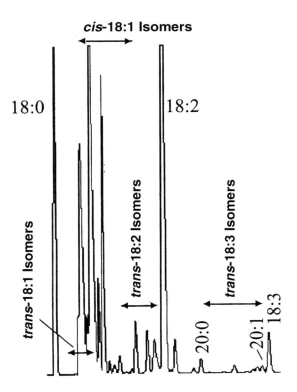

Fig. 4.9. Partial GC FAME profile (18:0 to 18:3) reported in AOCS method Ce 1f-96 for partially hydrogenated soybean oil using a 50-m CP-Sil 88 column (Reproduced by permission from AOCS Press).

ed by the thickness of the spacer (up to 1.00 mm), and the concentration of the absorbing analyte (c). To determine the amount of an unknown, (a) is first calculated by generating a plot of the absorbance of calibration standards (e.g., carbon disulfide (CS2) solutions of methyl elaidate) at different concentrations over the range of interest. When the analyte is a neat fat or oil (without solvent), the thickness of the spacer should be below 10 μm for the transmitted infrared radiation to reach the detector. This very short pathlength limitation is easily met by using ATR sampling techniques (Harrick, 1967; Internal Reflection Spectroscopy, 1992; Ismail *et al.*, 1998).

Attenuated Total Reflection Mode. When melted fat or oil is placed on the surface of a crystal such as diamond, the infrared light penetrates a distance of only a few μm into the test sample when the conditions of total internal reflection apply (Harrick, 1967; Internal Reflection Spectroscopy, 1992; Ismail *et al.*, 1998). These conditions occur when light traveling in a transparent medium of high refractive index (η_1) (such as diamond or ZnSe) strikes the interface between this medium and another transparent medium of lower refractive index (η_2) (such as air or melted *trans* fat) at an angle of incidence (θ) exceeding the critical angle (θ_c) defined by

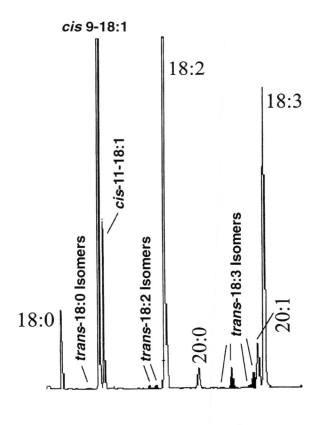

cis 9-18:1

18:2

18:3

18:0

trans-18:0 Isomers

cis-11-18:1

trans-18:2 Isomers

20:0

trans-18:3 Isomers

20:1

Fig. 4.10. Partial GC FAME profile (18:0 to 18:3) reported in AOCS method Ce 1f-96 (AOCS, 1999) for refined rapeseed oil using a 50-m CP-Sil 88 column (Reproduced by permission from AOCS Press).

$$\theta_c = \sin^{-1} (\eta_2/\eta_1)$$

Normally, light is partially transmitted and partially reflected. However, under these conditions, it is not transmitted, but totally reflected inside the crystal (Fig. 4.14). Moreover, as the light bounces (one or more times) inside the crystal, a so-called evanescent wave also propagates away from the surface of the crystal through the melted *trans* fat (Adam *et al.*, 2000; Mossoba *et al.*, 2001), in this example. At the surface of the crystal, the intensity of this wave decays exponentially with distance. It is also attenuated by the absorption of infrared light by the melted *trans* fat. The depth of penetration (d_p) of the infrared light into the test sample is minuscule. It typically varies between 1–4 μm and depends on θ, η_2, η_1, and the wavelength (λ) as given by the relation:

$$dp = \lambda/2 \, \pi \, \eta_1 \, [\sin^2 (\theta) - (\eta_2/\eta_1)]^{1/2}$$

As a result, the depth of penetration (which is also the effective pathlength) will be higher the greater λ or the smaller the frequency. Therefore, an interferogram (raw

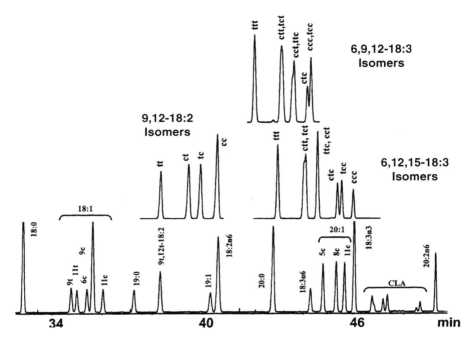

Fig. 4.11. A partial GC FAME profile (18:0 to 20:2n-6) of the FAME standard #463 spiked with the CLA mixture #UC-59M, both from Nu-Chek Prep. The mixtures of linoleic (9,12-18:2), γ-linolenic (9,12,15-18:3) and α-linolenic acid (6,9,12–18:3) isomers are placed above the lower chromatogram in the appropriate elution positions. A 100-m CP-Sil 88 column was used, and a temperature program from 45 to 215°C (Kramer *et al.*, 2002; Kramer *et al.*, 2001). (Reproduced by permission from AOCS Press).

infrared spectrum) is a measure of the attenuation by a *trans* fat test sample of the totally internally reflected infrared light. The interferogram of a reference background material (e.g., a *trans*-free fat) is similarly measured. They are subsequently used to obtain an absorption spectrum as explained above. ATR-FTIR measurements are easy, convenient, and require about 2 min per test sample (Adam *et al.*, 2000; Mossoba *et al.*, 2001).

Trans Fat Infrared Methodology. Because of the interest in accurate and rapid analytical methods for quantifying total *trans* fatty acids with isolated double bonds, many infrared spectroscopic procedures and official methods have been published over the past several decades (Mossoba *et al.*, 1996). These proposed procedures and official methods that have been validated through national and/or international multi-laboratory collaborative studies provide varying degrees of accuracy and reproducibility. A review is given below following an introduction about the scope of this infrared determination.

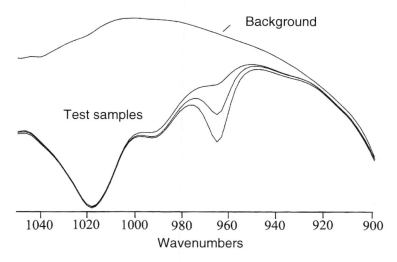

Fig. 4.12. Single-beam spectra for carbon disulfide (CS2) solvent (background) and CS2 solutions of *trans* fat (test samples).

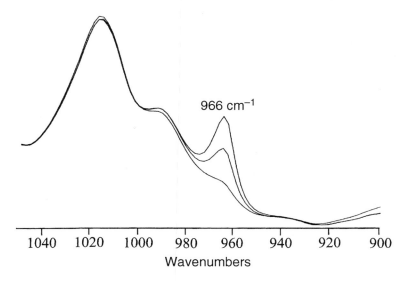

Fig. 4.13. Absorption spectra for CS2 solutions of *trans* fat (test samples).

The determination of total *trans* fatty acids by the different IR spectroscopic procedures (Mossoba *et al.*, 1996) and official methods (AOCS, 1999b; AOAC International, 1997a; AOCS, 1999c; AOAC International, 1997b) is based on the C-H out-of-plane deformation band observed at 966 cm^{-1} (Fig. 4.13) that is uniquely characteristic of isolated double bonds with *trans* configuration. These double bonds

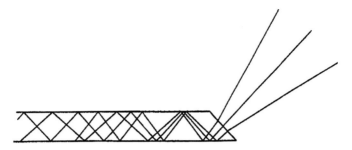

Fig. 4.14. Infrared light bouncing inside an internal reflection crystal.

are found primarily in *trans*-monoenes, and usually at much lower levels in minor hydrogenation products, such as methylene-interrupted (e.g., *trans* 9,*trans* 12-18:2) and nonmethylene-interrupted (e.g., *trans* 9,*trans* 13-18:2) *trans*,*trans*-dienes, mono-*trans*dienes (e.g., *trans* 9,*cis* 12-18:2), and other *trans*-polyenes. This IR methodology has been extensively used in the fats and oils industry and found to be extremely useful to determine the triacylglycerols or fatty acid methyl esters. However, samples consisting of free fatty acids must be first esterified particularly at low *trans* levels (less than 15%) (Firestone and Sheppard, 1992) because the band near 935 cm^{-1}, due to the O-H out-of plane deformation in –C(O)OH moieties would interfere with the determination of the *trans* band at 966 cm^{-1}.

When the total isolated *trans* fat levels are relatively low (below 10%), a potentially significant interference is found in products containing approximately 1% (such as milk fat) or more of conjugated unsaturation ((Firestone and Sheppard, 1992; Mossoba *et al.*, 2001a; Firestone and LaBouliere, 1965). This is due to the fact that conjugated *trans*,*trans* (near 990 cm^{-1}) and/or *cis*/*trans* (near 990 and 950 cm^{-1}) double bonds exhibit absorption bands that are sufficiently close to, and thus interfere with, the 966 cm^{-1} band. An analytical solution to this problem based on standard addition has been published (Mossoba *et al.*, 2001a). This procedure was recently used to determine the *trans* content of milkfat in the presence of interfering CLA isomers (Mossoba *et al.*, 2001a).

The highly characteristic *trans* absorption at 966 cm^{-1} occurs on an elevated and sloping baseline, thus the measurement of its height or area becomes increasingly less accurate as the *trans* levels decrease (Fig. 4.13). Since the early report by Firestone and LaBouliere (AOAC International, 1994) that the IR determination of *trans* unsaturation yielded a high bias for triacylglycerols and a low bias for fatty acid methyl esters, many modifications have been proposed. Transmission (AOCS, 1999b; AOAC International, 1997a) and internal reflection (AOCS, 1999c; AOAC International , 1997b) FTIR official methods succeeded in improving the accuracy of this determination.

Transmission FTIR Official Method AOCS Cd 14-95/AOAC 965.34. The latest transmission infrared official methods (AOCS, 1999b; AOAC International, 1997a) were improvements of older ones. It requires the analysis of all samples as fatty acid methyl esters (FAME) irrespective of *trans* level. FAME test samples are accurately weighed and dissolved in known volumes of CS2. FAME solutions are then measured by FTIR in 1-mm fixed-pathlength non-demountable transmission cells. FAME calibration standards each consisting of a known mixture of methyl elaidate and methyl oleate in CS2 were prepared, such that the total concentration of FAMEs was the same (0.2 g/10 mL) for all standards. The total concentration of test samples was also set at 0.2 g/10 mL. This method assumes that the major component to be determined in test samples is methyl elaidate. Two linear regression calibration equations were generated, one for the set of standards with *trans* contents of ≤10% and another for those with *trans* levels >10%. To measure the 966-cm^{-1} band height, a straight line was first drawn between two points along the sloping baseline of the infrared spectrum (Fig. 4.13). The positions of these two points were determined by the analyst, and had to be moved closer to each other as the size of the *trans* band decreased. Validation data generated in multi-laboratory studies using this and other infrared official methods will be compared below.

ATR-FTIR Official Method AOCS Cd 14d-99/AOAC 2000.10. Using internal reflection, also known as attenuated total reflection (ATR), another official method (AOCS, 1999c; AOAC International , 1997b) was recently developed to rapidly (5 min) measure the 966-cm^{-1} *trans* band as a symmetric feature on a *horizontal* baseline. The experimental aspects of this ATR infrared official method are far less complex than those involving transmission measurements. This approach uses "ratioing" the *trans* test sample single-beam spectrum against that of a reference material consisting of a *trans*-free oil and applies the ATR sampling technique (Harrick, 1967; Internal Reflection Spectroscopy, 1992; Ismail *et al.*, 1998; Adam *et al.*, 2000; Mossoba *et al.*, 2001) to melted fats; this avoids the weighing of test portions and their quantitative dilution with the volatile CS2 solvent.

In today's FTIR instruments (Reedy and Mossoba 1999), single beam spectra are measured separately for both a test sample and an appropriate reference background material, and then "ratioed" to obtain an absorption spectrum. Traditionally, CS2 solvent has been used as the reference background material in the vast majority of procedures and official methods (Mossoba *et al.*, 1996; AOCS, 1999b; AOAC Interntional, 1997a). When a *trans*-free fat reference background material is used (Fig. 4.15) instead of CS2, the sloping baseline of the 966 cm^{-1} *trans* band (Fig. 4.13) becomes horizontal (Fig. 4.16) (Adam *et al.*, 2000; Mossoba *et al.*, 2001; Mossoba *et al.*, 1996). Therefore, the contributions of the triacylglycerol absorptions that led to the sloping baseline in the first place are removed, and the requirement to convert triacylglycerols to FAME is eliminated.

Having a horizontal baseline minimizes the uncertainty in the measurement of the 966 cm^{-1} *trans* band area at all *trans* levels, and improves both precision and accuracy. This approach of using a *trans*-free reference background material can be used in both transmission or internal reflection modes. In transmission mode, a CS2 solution

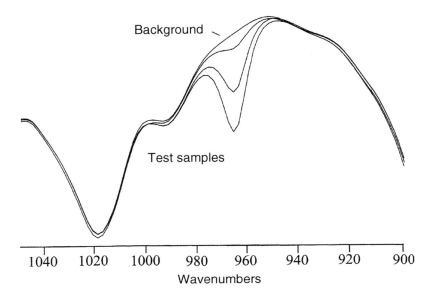

Fig. 4.15. Single-beam spectra for neat (without solvent) *trans*-free fat (background) and *trans* fat (test samples).

of the test sample is "ratioed" against a CS2 solution of a *trans*-free reference background material, or simply a neat (without solvent) test sample is "ratioed" against a neat *trans*-free reference background material. The latter is easily and rapidly achieved with an ATR cell as described by the official method and explained next.

Accurately weighed *trans* standards are prepared by adding varying amounts (0–50%) of neat trielaidin to a neat *trans*-free reference oil. Next, a small volume of a standard is placed on top of the heated (65°C) horizontal surface of the internal reflection element (usually zinc selenide or diamond) of a single-bounce ATR cell. Depending on the size of the internal reflection element, this small volume can range from 50 μL to as little as 1 μL. The element surface must be completely covered. Single beam spectra (Fig. 4.15) of *trans* standards (test samples) are measured by FTIR and "ratioed" against the single beam spectrum of the same *trans*free reference oil (background) to obtain absorption spectra. These spectra should exhibit the 966-cm^{-1} *trans* band as a symmetric feature on a horizontal baseline (Fig. 4.16). The areas of the *trans* bands can then be integrated electronically between 990 and 945 cm^{-1} and used to generate a calibration curve. The resulting linear regression equation relating the integrated area and the *trans* level (as percent of total fat) of the standards usually has a negligible y-intercept and a regression coefficient R value of 0.999 (Adam *et al.*, 2000; Mossoba *et al.*, 2001; AOCS, 1999c, AOAC International, 1997b).

Similarly, single beam spectra of unknown *trans* test samples are measured and "ratioed" against the single beam spectrum of the same *trans*-free reference oil used for calibration. The *trans* level (as percent of total fat) is then calculated by substitut-

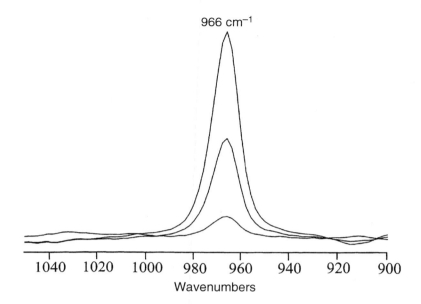

Fig. 4.16. Absorption spectra for neat (without solvent) *trans* fat (test samples).

ing the value of the integrated area of the *trans* band in the linear regression equation. This method also assumes that the major component to be determined in test samples is trielaidin.

The fatty acid composition of the *trans*-free reference oil plays a critical role. If the selected *trans*-free oil is significantly different from the matrix of the fat investigated, it may have an adverse impact on accuracy, particularly near the official method's lowest *trans* level of quantitation, 5%, as percent of total fat. This *trans*-free reference oil must be carefully selected and should resemble as much as possible the composition of the unknown *trans* fat or oil being determined.

When the corresponding FAME were used instead of triacylglycerols, similar *trans* values were obtained (Mossoba *et al.*, 1996), thus demonstrating that this "ratioing" ATR FTIR method adequately compensates for the triacylglycerol absorptions that overlap with the 966-cm^{-1} *trans* band and contribute to its elevated and sloping baseline. In comparative studies, lower reproducibility relative standard deviation, RSD(R), values (Adam, 2000; Mossoba, 2001) were obtained by using the ATR-FTIR method (AOCS, 1999c, AOAC International, 1997b) relative to two transmission FTIR methods (AOCS, 1999b; AOAC International, 1997a; Griinari *et al.*, 2000) (Fig. 4.17).

Present Status and Limitations of Official Methods

The determination of fatty acid composition and total *trans* fat by a single GC run has been the industry standard (Wolff and Precht, 2002; Precht and Molkentin, 1999;

Pariza *et al.*, 2001; Kramer *et al.*, 2002; Kramer *et al.*, 2001; Buchgraber and Ulberth, 2001). These determinations became easier with the availability of 100 m highly polar capillary columns. Efforts are presently underway at the AOCS to modify the official GC method for *trans* fatty acid determination using the 100 m highly polar capillary GC columns. However, this task still requires extensive expertise in identifying all possible *trans*-containing fatty acids and their isomers, many of which remain unresolved and overlap with other fatty acids (Wolff and Precht, 2002; Precht *et al.*, 2001; Cruz-Hernandez *et al.*, 2004). Depending on the column used and the sample analyzed, the total *trans* content may be underestimated by as much as 35% (Precht *et al.*, 2001). Accurate determinations require the combination of a preliminary silver-ion chromatographic (TLC or HPLC) separation of *trans* from *cis* geometric isomers (5-Wolff, 1995; Henninger and Ulberth, 1994; Kramer *et al.*, 2002; Kramer *et al.*, 2001; Precht *et al.*, 2001; Cruz-Hernandez *et al.*, 2004) followed by a low temperature isothermal GC analysis. The ideal chromatographic methodology

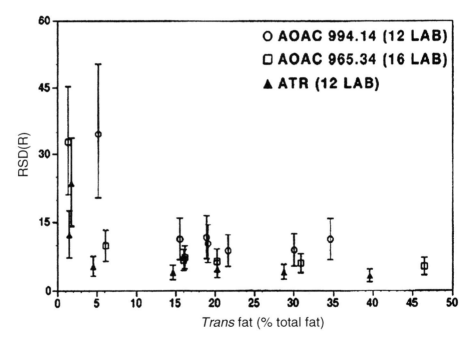

Fig. 4.17. Comparison of plots of reproducibility relative standard deviation, RSD(R), against the *trans* content mean values determined by three official methods: the two transmission methods AOAC 965.34 and AOAC 994.14, and the ATR method AOCS Cd 14d-99. The number of laboratories in the corresponding collaborative studies were 12,16, and 12, respectively. The error bars denote the upper and lower 95% confidence limits on the true RSD(R). (Reproduced by permission from AOCS Press).

for the quantitation of *trans* fatty acids has yet to be developed and validated. GC official methods do not state lower levels of quantitation, but they have been generally used to determine *trans* levels as low as 0.5%, as percent of total fat.

At the present time the proposed *trans* regulations in Canada (http://canadagazette, 2003) and the US (DHHS, 2003) do not require a distinction between the different *trans* fatty acid isomers. However, the need to separate the different *trans* fatty acid isomers may become necessary if findings are confirmed that certain *trans* isomers have nutritionally and/or physiologically desirable properties. Specifically, the *trans* 11-18:1 isomer was reported to be a precursor for CLA production in mammalian tissues (Griinari *et al.*, 2000; Bauman and Griinari, 2001) and CLA isomers have been reported to have beneficial physiological effects in many animal models (Pariza *et al.*, 2001). In this case, the GC method will become an essential research tool.

Infrared spectroscopy has been the tool of choice for the rapid determination of *total* isolated *trans* double bonds in oils and fats (AOCS, 1999b; AOAC, 1997a). The new ATR-FTIR official method (AOCS, 1999e; AOAC, 1997b) can be applied conveniently to the determination of the total *trans* content of fats in the vast majority of food products. FTIR official methods are only applicable to food products containing more than 5% *trans*, as percent of total fat (AOAC, 1997b). It was recently reported that by using the negative second derivative (−2D) instead of the absorption spectrum itself, spectral features were enhanced such that *trans* fatty acid levels as low as 0.5% could be readily measured (Milosevic *et al.*, 2004). The FTIR methods are more rapid than GC methods, but do not provide detailed information on fatty acid composition. Although for *trans* fatty acid nutrition labeling, information regarding *trans* isomeric distributions is currently not required, the exclusion of CLA is (DHHS, 2003). Differentiation of the *trans* absorption band attributed to CLA isomers containing a conjugated *trans* bond from that of isolated *trans* fatty acids remains a challenge (Kramer *et al.*, 1997). The total *trans* content can be measured independently using a standard addition technique based on the IR measurement of trielaidin (Mossoba *et al.*, 2001a), or resolving the IR absorption bands by using second derivative FTIR spectra (Milosevic *et al.*, 2004).

Recent advances in Fourier transform-near infrared (FT-NIR) have made it possible to determine not only the total *trans* fatty acid content of a fat or oil as by ATR-FTIR, but also its fatty acid composition (Azizian *et al.*, 2004), and without the need for prior derivatization to volatile derivatives as required for GC analysis. Quantitative FT-NIR models were developed by comparing accurate GC results with FT-NIR measurements and using chemometric analyses. FT-NIR has also been applied to the determination of CLA in the presence of *trans* fatty acids (Christy *et al.*, 2003). FT-NIR methodologies show great potential, but they will need to be validated in collaborative studies.

In addition, there is a specific need to address differences in total *trans* fatty acid content that are obtained by chromatographic and spectroscopic techniques. This problem may perhaps be related to unidentified *trans* fatty acid GC peaks, non-lipid *trans* infrared absorptions, or to the nature of specific food matrices. Consistencies between GC and FTIR methods will need to be validated for accuracy, reliability and applicability to different foods.

References

Adam, M., Mossoba, M.M., and Lee, T., Rapid Determination of Total *trans* Fat Content by Attenuated Total Reflection Infrared Spectroscopy: An International Collaborative Study, *J. Am. Oil Chem. Soc. 77:*457–462 (2000).

AOAC International, Method 994.14, *Official Methods of Analysis, 16th edition*, Gaithersburg, MD, 1994.

AOAC International, Method 996.06, revised 2001, *Official Methods of Analysis,* 17th edition, Gaithersburg, MD, 1997.

AOAC International, Method 965.34, *Official Methods of Analysis, 17th edition*, Gaithersburg, MD, 1997a.

AOAC International, Method 2000.10, *Official Methods of Analysis, 17th edition*, Gaithersburg, MD, 1997b

AOCS, Official Method Ce 1f-96, revised 2002, *American Oil Chemists' Society, Official Methods and Recommended Practices,* 5th edition, ed., Firestone, D., Champaign, IL, 1999.

AOCS, Official Method Ce 1g-96, *American Oil Chemists' Society, Official Methods and Recommended Practices*, 5th edition, ed., Firestone, D., Champaign, IL, 1999a.

AOCS, Official Method Cd 14-95, *American Oil Chemists' Society, Official Methods and Recommended Practices*, 5th edition, ed., Firestone, D., Champaign, IL, 1999b.

AOCS, Official Method Cd 14d-99, *American Oil Chemists' Society, Official Methods and Recommended Practices, 5th edition*, ed., Firestone, D., Champaign, IL, 1999c.

Azizian, H., Winsborough, S.L., Kramer, J.K.G., Hernandez, M. and Mossoba, M.M., Quantification of *Trans* Fatty Acids in Foods by GC, ATR-FTIR and FT-NIR Methods, *Lipid Technol. 16*, 229-231 (2004).

Bauman, D.E., and Griinari, J.M., Regulation and Nutritional Manipulation of Milk Fat: Low-Fat Milk Syndrome, *Livestock Prod. Sci. 70:*15–29 (2001).

Buchgraber, M., and Ulberth, F., Determination of *trans* Octadecenoic Acids by Silver-Ion Chromatography-Gas Liquid Chromatography: An Intercomparison of Methods, *AOAC International 84:*1490–1498 (2001).

Chardigny, J.-M., Wolff, R.L., Mager, E., Bayard, C.C., Sébédio, J.-L., Martine, L., and Ratnayake, W.M.N. Fatty Acid Composition of French Infant Formulas with Emphasis on the Content and Detailed Profile of *trans* Fatty Acids, *J. Am. Oil Chem. Soc. 73:*1595–1601 (1996).

Christy, A. A., Egeberg, P.K., Ostensen, E.T., Simultaneous quantitative determination of isolated trans fatty acids and conjugated linoleic acids in oils and fats by chemometric analysis of the infrared profiles, *Vibrational Spectroscopy 33,* 37-48 (2003).

Craig-Schmidt, M.C. Consumption of *trans* Fatty Acids in *trans Fatty Acids in Human Nutrition*, eds. J.L. Sébédio and W.W. Christie, The Oily Press, Dundee, Scotland, 1998, pp. 59–114.

Cruz-Hernandez, C. Deng, Z. Zhou, J. Hill, A.R., Yurawecz, M.P., Delmonte, P., Mossoba, M.M., Dugan, M.E.R. Kramer, J.K.G., Methods to Analyze Conjugated Linoleic Acids (CLA) and *Trans*-18:1 Isomers in Dairy Fats Using a Combination of GC, Silver Ion TLC-GC, and Silver Ion HPLC, *J. AOAC International 87*, 545-562 (2004).

Department of Health and Human Services, FDA (2003) Food Labeling; *Trans* Fatty Acids in Nutrition Labeling; Nutrient Content Claims, and Health Claims; Final Rule, *Federal Register 68*, No. 133, July 11, 2003, pp.41434-41506.

Duchateau, G.S.M.J.E., van Osten, H.J., and Vasconcellos, M.A., Analysis of *cis-* and *trans-* fatty Acid Isomers in Hydrogenated and Refined Vegetable Oils by Capillary Gas–liquid Chromatography, *J. Am. Oil Chem. Soc. 73*:273–278 (1996).

Firestone, D., and LaBouliere, P., Determination of Isolated *trans* Isomers by Infrared Spectrophotometry, *J. Assoc. Off. Anal. Chem. Vol. 48*:437–443 (1965).

Firestone, D., and Sheppard, A., Determination of *trans* fatty acids, in *Advances in Lipid Methodology-One*, W.W. Christie (editor), The Oily Press, Ayr, UK, 1992, pp. 273–322.

Fritsche, J., and Steinhart, H. *Analysis of trans* Fatty Acids in *New Trends in Lipid Analysis*, eds. M.M. Mossoba and R.E. McDonald, AOCS Press, Champaign, Illinois, 1997, pp. 234–256.

Griinari, J.M., Corl, B.A., Lacy, S.H., Chouinard, P.Y., Nurmela, K.V.V. and Bauman, D.E., Conjugated Linoleic Acid is Synthesized Endogenously in Lactating Dairy Cows by ?^{9}-Desaturase, *J. Nutr. 130*, 2285-2291 (2000)

Harrick, N.J., *Internal Reflection Spectroscopy*, Wiley-Interscience, New York, NY, 1967.

Henninger, M., and Ulberth, F., *trans* Fatty Acid Content of Bovine Milk Fat, *Milchwissenschaft 49*:555–558 (1994).

http://canadagazette.gc.ca/partII/2003/20030101/html/sor11-e.html.

Internal Reflection Spectroscopy, *Practical Spectroscopy Series, Vol. 15*, ed., Mirabella, F.M., Marcel Dekker, New York, NY, 1992.

Ismail, A.A., Nicodemo, A., Sedman, J., van de Voort, F.R., and Holzbauer, I.E., Infrared Spectroscopy of Lipids: Principles and Applications in *Spectral Properties of Lipids*, ed., Hamilton, R.J., and Cast, J., Sheffield Academic Press/CRC Press, Boca Raton, FL, pp. 235–269, 1998.

Kramer, J.K.G., Blackadar, C.B., and Zhou, J., Evaluation of Two GC Columns (60-m Supelcowax 10 and 100-m CP Sil 88) for Analysis of Milkfat with Emphasis on CLA, 18:1, 18:2, and 18:3 Isomers, and Short- and Long-Chain FA, *Lipids, 37*:823–835 (2002).

Kramer, J.K.G., Cruz-Hernandez, C., and Zhou, J., Conjugated Linoleic Acids and Octadecenoic Acids: Analysis by GC. *Eur. J. Lipid Sci. Technol. 103:*600–609 (2001).

Kramer, J.K.G., Feller, V., Dugan, M.E.R., Sauer, F.D., Mossoba, M.M., and Yurawecz, M.P., Evaluating Acid and Base Catalysts in the Methylation of Milk and Rumen Fatty Acids with Special Emphasis on Conjugated Dienes and Total *trans* Fatty Acids, *Lipids 32*:1219–1228 (1997).

Milosevic, M., Milosovic, V., Kramer, J.K.G., Azizian, H. and Mossoba, M.M., Determining Low Levels of *Trans* Fatty Acids in Foods by an Improved Atr-ftir Procedure, *Lipid Technol. 16*, 229-231 (2004).

Mossoba, M.M., Adam, M., and Lee, T., Rapid Determination of Total *trans* Fat Content. An Attenuated Total Reflection Infrared Spectroscopy International Collaborative Study, *AOAC International, 84:*1144–1150 (2001).

Mossoba, M.M., Kramer, J.K.G., Fritsche, J., Yurawecz, M.P., Eulitz, K., Ku, Y., and Rader, J.I., Application of Standard Addition to Eliminate Conjugated Linoleic Acid and Other Interferences in the Determination of Total *trans*

Mossoba, M.M., Yurawecz, M.P., and McDonald, R.E., Rapid Determination of the Total *trans* Content of Neat Hydrogenated Oils by Attenuated Total Reflection Spectroscopy, *J. Am. Oil Chem. Soc. 73*:1003–1009, (1996), and references therein.

Pariza, M.P., Park, Y., and Cook, M.E., The Biologically Active Isomers of Conjugated Linoleic Acid, *Progr. Lipid Res. 40:*283–298 (2001).

Precht, D., and Molkentin, J., C18:1, C18:2 and C18:3 trans and cis Fatty Acid Isomers Including Conjugated cis-9,trans-11 Linoleic Acid (CLA) as well as Total Fat Composition of German Human Milk Lipids, Nahrung 43:233–244 (1999).

Precht, D., and Molkentin, J., Frequency Distribution of Conjugated Linoleic Acid and trans Fatty Acid Contents in European Bovine Milk Fats, Milchwissenschaft 55:687–691 (2000).

Precht, D., Molkentin, J., Destaillats, F. and Wolff, R.L., Comparative Studies on Individual Isomeric 18:1 Acids in Cows, Goats, and Ewe Milk Fats by low-Temperature High-Resolution Capillary Gs-Liquid Chromatography, Lipids, 36, 827-832 (2001).

Ratnayake, W.M.N., Analysis of Dietary trans Fatty Acids, J. Oleo Sci. 50:73–86 (2001).

Reedy, G., and Mossoba, M.M., Matrix Isolation GC-FTIR, in Spectral Methods in Food Analysis, ed. Mossoba, M.M., Marcel Dekker, Inc., New York, NY, pp. 325–396, 1999.

Wolff, R.L., Content and Distribution of trans-18:1 Acids in Ruminant Milk and Meat Fats. Their Importance in European Diets and Their Effects on Human Milk, J. Am. Oil Chem. Soc. 72:259–272 (1995).

Wolff, R.L., and Precht, D. A Critique of 50-m CP-Sil 88 Capillary Columns Used Alone to Assess trans-Unsaturated FA in Foods: The Case of TRANSFAIR Study, Lipids 37:627–629 (2002).

Wolff RL, Precht D, Molkentin J. Occurrence and Distribution Profiles of trans-18:1 Acids in Edible Fats of Natural Origin in trans Fatty Acids in Human Nutrition, eds. J.L. Sébédio and W.W. Christie, The Oily Press, Dundee, Scotland, 1998, pp. 1–34.

Yurawecz, M.P., Roach, J.A.G., Sehat, N., Mossoba, M.M., Kramer, J.K.G., Fritsche, J., Steinhart, H., and Ku, Y., A New Conjugated Linoleic Acid Isomer, 7 trans, 9 cisTrans Octadecadienoic Acid, in Cow Milk, Cheese, Beef and Human Milk, and Adipose Tissue, Lipids 33:803–809 (1998).

Chapter 5

Dietary Guidelines, Processing, and Reformulation for *Trans* Reduction

G. R. List[1] and Robert Reeves[2]

[1]Food and Industrial Oil Research, National Center for Agricultural Utilization Research, Agricultural Research Service, U.S. Department of Agriculture, 1815 N. University Street, Peoria, IL 61604, listgr@ncaur.usda.gov;
[2]Institute of Shortening and Edible Oils, Washington, D.C. 20006

Introduction

In 1990, the United States Congress passed the Nutrition Labeling and Education Act (NLEA). The Food and Drug Administration (FDA) established regulations in 1993 pursuant to NLEA basically revising the mandatory information required on food labels. The main elements of these regulations were nutrition labeling, nutrient content descriptors and health messages. In November, 1999, FDA proposed regulations which would include *trans* fat in the "saturated fat" column of the nutrition facts panel of food labels. However, on November 15, 2002, FDA revised its proposed rule on trans fat labeling by proposing to declare *trans* fat individually in the nutrition facts panel and link it to a footnote stating "Intake of *trans* fat should be as low as possible." The final regulation was announced on July 11, 2003 which required a quantitative declaration of *trans* fat in the nutrition facts panel, however no footnote was required nor were nutrient content claims (e.g., "no *trans* fat," "reduced *trans* fat") approved at this time. Foods containing less than 0.5g *trans* fat per serving must declare the amount as "0." No percent daily value (%DV) was established for *trans* fats due to a lack of scientific information. The effective date of the rule was January 1, 2006. This chapter will review the methods by which the food industry is reformulating foods in order to reduce *trans* fats in the U.S. diet, be in compliance with FDA's regulation, and provide foods that are consistent with the U.S. Dietary Guidelines for Americans, 2005.

Dietary Guidelines

The Dietary Guidelines for Americans 2005 were jointly announced on 1-12-05 by the Departments of Health and Human Sciences (HHS) and Agriculture (USDA) (Anon 2005). These guidelines have been updated every five years since 1975 as a means for health, nutrition and medical professionals to provide advice to Americans regarding the promotion of health and reducing the risk of chronic disease through nutrition and physical activity.

The Dietary Guidelines offer recommendations in several important areas including weight management, physical activity, food safety and consumption of macronutrients (e.g., fat, carbohydrates, and protein). Although dietary fat management is addressed in the Dietary Guidelines, this chapter will focus particularly on the current actions being taken by the food industry to reduce *trans* fat in the diet.

The Dietary Guidelines 2005 make the following recommendations on fat consumption: (i) consume less than 10% calories from saturated fats and less than 300 mg/d of cholesterol and keep *trans* fat consumption as low as possible; (ii) keep total fat intake between 20-35% of calories (mostly poly- and monounsaturated fats); (iii) make meat, poultry, dry bean and milk product choices "lean," "low fat," or "fat free;" and (iv) limit intakes of fats and oils high in saturated and/or *trans* fats.

In making its recommendations on dietary fat intake, the Dietary Guidelines authors reviewed many recent scientific documents and studies. Perhaps one of the more important scientific references used in guiding the establishment of the Dietary Guidelines, 2005 is the Institute of Medicine/National Academies of Science Report on Macronutrients, published September 5, 2002 (Anon 2002). It states "most Americans need to decrease their intakes of saturated fat and *trans* fats, and many need to decrease their dietary intake of cholesterol." The report further points out that the food industry has an important role in decreasing *trans* fat content in foods since about 80% are accounted for in foods containing partially hydrogenated oils while the remaining 20% are supplied by ruminant animals (i.e., beef and dairy products).

Trans Fat Reduction in Foods/Oils

The reduction of *trans* fats in foods has been influenced by many factors. One major factor is FDA's *trans* fat labeling regulation, which will require the inclusion of *trans* fats within the nutrition facts panel of the food label by 1-1-06 (Anon 2003). The agency is also considering the use of nutrient content claims such as "*trans* fat free" and "reduced *trans* fat" to further guide consumers in their choice of foods.

The food industry is also assuming its responsibility to the American public by providing them with more healthful foods that can fit into a daily diet. American consumers are becoming more health conscious and are increasingly interested in food products of increased healthfulness. Consumer advocacy groups have also called for the labeling of *trans* fats and their reduction in the diet.

The attempts by the food industry to reduce dietary *trans* fats have largely resulted in food manufacturers seeking reformulated food ingredients that are lower or devoid of *trans* fat. Restaurants are similarly switching to deep frying oils with reduced *trans* fat. Some retail food markets have even attempted to market only foods containing "low" or "no" *trans* fats.

Challenges

There are many challenges that food manufacturers have faced during the development of new *trans* fat alternatives. Any replacement ingredient must provide the functional characteristics of the material being replaced. In other words, the alternative ingredient must provide the functionality of flakiness, firmness of texture, crispness or desired appearance in the finished product or it is likely to be rejected by the consumer. The stability or shelf life of the finished product must also be maintained to ensure consumer acceptability.

Another major factor involved in the development of *trans* fat alternatives is the assurance that such products will be available in adequate commercial quantities. For example, a major restaurant chain must be assured that any new food product or frying medium will be available in sufficient quantities to satisfy anticipated demand. In some cases, this may mean very large commercial quantities. Similarly suppliers of *trans* fat alternatives (e.g., vegetable oils derived from oilseed varieties having unique fatty acid profiles) may require commitments from restaurant chains or food manufacturers to purchase sufficient amounts of the alternative ingredient to justify the major capital investment necessary to bring the alternative product to the marketplace. Newer oilseed varieties containing oil of increased stability, thus having less need for partial hydrogenation, may take six to seven years to commercially develop in a best-case scenario.

Alternatives to Hydrogenation

There are currently four main sources of *trans* fat alternatives: naturally stable oils/fats, interesterified oils, "modified" partially hydrogenated oils and trait-enhanced oils from newer oilseed varieties.

The more common oils or fats that are relatively stable and requiring little or no partial hydrogenation for most food product applications thus containing no *trans* fats include palm, corn and cottonseed oils. Also used to a lesser extent are palm kernel, coconut, high oleic canola, high oleic safflower, mid and high oleic sunflower, and low linolenic soybean oils as well as animal fats.

A second source of relatively stable oils is through the use of oils that have undergone the process of "interesterification." This process rearranges the fatty acids in a fat molecule resulting in customized melting characteristics.

A third method that may be used to reduce *trans* fats is by modifying the process of partial hydrogenation. Alteration of the variables influencing the hydrogenation process (e.g., time, temperature, catalyst) can result in a partially hydrogenated product of significantly reduced *trans* fat content (List 2004a).

The fourth method of reducing *trans* fats in the diet is to use oils from "trait enhanced" oilseed varieties specifically designed to have increased stability. These newer oilseed varieties are usually bred to have either lower amounts of relatively unstable fatty acids (e.g., linolenic) or higher amounts of more stable fatty acids (e.g., oleic). Such oilseed varieties currently available or soon to be introduced commercially include mid oleic sunflower and soybean, low linolenic soybean and canola, and high oleic sunflower and canola. Such varieties may be derived from either traditional plant breeding practices or biotechnological methods.

The newer technologies required to develop many *trans* fat alternatives are relatively expensive. These costs are likely to be passed on to consumers in the form of higher food prices. If foods become too expensive, consumers may not purchase them regardless of their nutritional value or functionality.

Another challenge to suppliers of *trans* fat alternatives is the logistics of physically providing them to end users. There is no single solution to solving food manufacturer needs in a variety of products. Multiple ingredient alternatives require multiple inventories and often times multiple suppliers. Also a major source of a *trans* fat alternative may be limited to only one or perhaps a few regional supply sources, placing major demands on supply systems attempting to service geographically diverse and numerous receivers of such products. Significant "lead time" may be required from the time of ordering to the time of delivery.

The search for oils that may be used in *trans* fat alternative products has had certain effects on the edible oils marketplace. Palm oil imports in 2003-04 were about 220,000 metric tons, in 2004-05 they were about 408,200 metric tons (375,000 in food use), and estimates are that about 600,000 metric tons will be imported in 2005-06. Other relatively stable oils that will be available in commercial quantities in the future include low linolenic soybean (2005-2008), low linolenic, mid oleic soybean (2009-2012), high stearic soybean (2008-2012) and high stearic canola (2008-2012). Low linolenic acid soybeans are expected to be the next variety of significant consequence with about 80 million pounds of oil available by fall of 2005 and about 2 billion pounds available in 2008 (Anon 2004a). The mid oleic variety of soybean is expected to be commercially available in 2007 (40 million pounds) with an expected availability of 2 billion pounds by 2010.

In summary, the food industry has faced several major challenges in bringing to the marketplace acceptable food products that are lower in or free of *trans* fats. They include: (i) insuring the availability of *trans* fat replacements in adequate quantities to satisfy the marketplace, (ii) achieving the functional characteristics of the product being replaced (i.e., texture, crispness, appearance, stability), (iii) minimizing the costs of *trans* fat replacements, and (iv) managing the logistics of preparing *trans* fat replacements (e.g., utilizing existing manufacturing facilities) and delivering them efficiently to food processors. The food industry has been working diligently to meet these challenges in order to provide *trans* fat alternatives that will meet the objectives of the Dietary Guidelines 2005 and provide the desirable characteristics in many foods demanded by consumers. A variety of such products are currently available in the marketplace and many others are on the horizon.

Reformulation

A variety of processing methods are available to reduce the *trans* acid content of edible fats and oils including chemical/enzymatic interesterification, fractionation, modified hydrogenation, blending of hard and soft feed stocks and genetic/plant breeding techniques. These techniques may be used singly or in combination with each other.

Interesterification

A review of the interesterification process is beyond the scope of this chapter. The reader is referred to a recent review (Rozendall and MaCrae 1997). Aside from hydrogenation, interesterification is the oldest fat modification method used to prepare plastic fats and was practiced in the United States on a commercial scale in the 1950's to improve the crystal habits of lard. Today, this technology is highly developed in Europe and is used to prepare a wide variety of margarine/spreads, shortenings and baking fats.

Application to Zero/Low trans Spreads/Shortening Oils

The patent literature is replete with information on interesterification as a route to low *trans* fats and oils. An excellent resource covers the patent literature from 1960 to 1974 (Gillies 1974). A further search of the patent literature using margarine/shortening and interesterification as key words yields over 46,000 references since 1976 alone. Thus a comprehensive review would not be practical. A summary is shown in Table 5.1. Instead, several examples will be given from the author's laboratory. Random interesterification of 80% liquid soybean oil with 20% completely hydrogenated soybean oil provides a route to soft margarine oil having suitable solid fat and crystal structure (List *et al*. 1977). Further work, in which the interesterified oils were formulated into soft margarines in the pilot plant, demonstrated that the 80:20 blend produced margarine that was harder and more difficult to spread than hydrogenated controls but an additional 20% liquid oil was required in the formulation. The product had suitable spreadability, sensory properties and resistance to oil/water loss (List *et al*. 1995a).

Random interesterification of other liquid oils including corn, peanut, cottonseed, canola and palm oil with completely hydrogenated soybean or cottonseed flakes yields basestocks suitable for formulation of zero *trans* margarines and shortenings (List *et al*. 1995b).

Shortening oils require higher, flatter solid fat curves and melting points than margarine oils. In order to obtain these properties, it is necessary to incorporate more stearine with the interesterified blend. The desired solid fat and melting point points are achieved by blending the interesterified basestock with additional liquid oil. The effect is shown in Figure 5.1 where the solid fat indexes of a 50:50 mixture of interesterified soybean oil and soybean stearine (IV 0) are shown along with mixtures (5-50%) of the basestock and liquid oil. Typically, all-purpose shortening prepared from hydrogenated components show SFI values at 50, 70, 92 and 104°F of 18-23, 14-19, 13-14 and 7-11 respectively. The 50:50 blend of interesterified and liquid soybean oil closely match these values and the drop melting point of 42.2°C is close to the 45-47 value observed for commercial products. Fluid shortenings can be prepared by blending 35% of the basestock with 65% soybean, corn, peanut, cottonseed or canola oils.

Enzymatic Interesterification

Production of *trans*-free fats via enzyme catalyzed interesterification became a commercial reality in 2004 (Anon 2004b). The process involves passage of blended liq-

TABLE 5.1

U.S. Patents Relating to Interesterification, Partial Hydrogenation and Blending of Fats and Oils for Low/Zero *trans* Acids Products.

Subject	Oil Components	Inventor	Patent No.	Year
Margarine	Lauric acid oils	Lindsay	2,996,388	1961
Margarine	Lauric/non-lauric acid oils	Babayan	3,268,340	1966
Margarine	Long and short chain fatty acids	Sieden	3,353,964	1967
Margarine	Palm kernal oil	Galenkamp	3,210,197	1965
Margarine	Lauric acid oils	Sieden	3,592,661	1971
Margarine	High PUFA, low *trans*	Melnick	2,921,855	1960
Margarine	Cottonseed stearine	Gooding	3,099,564	1963
Margarine	Safflower, peanut oil	Schmidt	3,240,608	1966
Margarine	High PUFA	Westenberg	3,600,195	1971
Margarine	High PUFA, tropical oil	Fondu	3,634,100	1972
Margarine	High PUFA	McNaught	3,746,551	1973
Low calorie fats	Medium + long chain fatty acids	Sieden	5,288,512	1994
Shortening, filler fat	Hyd. oil, tallow, lard	Kidger	3,244,536	1966
Confectionary	Lauric acid oils, long chain alcohols	Brown	3,512,994	1970
Cake shortening	Lard, vegetable oil, itaconic acid	Gleason	2,966,412	1960
Cake shortening	Animal/vegetable fats, hydroxy carboxylic acids	Gleason	2,970,055	1961
Plastic shortening	Liquid oil, interesterified hardstock	Thompson	3,102,814	1963
All purpose shortening	Low *trans* hydrogenated oil, hardstock	Scavone	US95/02745	1995
Plastic shortening	Liquid oil, hyd. oil, esterified propoxylated glycerine	Mazurek	6,495,188	2002
All purpose shortening	Canola oil, hardstock	Robert	VS94/0594	1994
Cake shortening	Animal fats	Steffen	2,855,310	1958
Plastic shortening	Lard, palm oil, vegetable oils	Nelson	2,855,311	1958
Margarine	Low *trans*, High in PUFA	Melnick	2,921,855	1960
Cholesterol lowering spread	Palm, soy, canola, olive	Sundram	5,578,334	1996
Cholesterol lowering spread	Canola, hyd. soy	Mettenen	5,502,045	1996
Sterol fortified food	Sunflower, rapeseed, palm, palm kernal	Amerongon	6,117,475	2000
Margarine hardstock	Soy, canola, sunflower, palm, palm kernal	Huizinga	6,156,370	2000

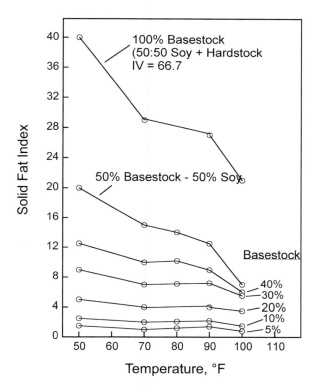

Fig. 5.1. Solid fat indexes of a 50:50 mixture of interesterified soybean oil and soybean stearine (IV 0), along with mixtures (5-50%) of the basestock and liquid oil.

uid oil and hardstock (IV = 0-5) in a ratio of 4:1 through a series of reactors holding an immobilized enzyme. Four reactors, holding from 100-400 kg of enzyme each, can produce 20-100 tons of fat per day. The enzyme is heat stable and may be reused and, since no side products are formed, no post processing is required. Both margarine and shortening bases are in the marketplace.

Fractionation

Rapid growth of the palm industry, beginning in the mid 1970's, prompted development of improved fractionation technology. Historically, solvent and detergent processes had been used, but today physical or dry fractionation is the industry standard. Palm oil (IV 51-53) is fractionated into olein (IV 56-59) and stearine fractions (IV 32-36). The olein fraction is further fractionated into mid-fractions and super oleins and top oleins. The palm mid fractions (IV 42-48) is further processed into harder fractions (IV 32-36. Fractionation of the stearine (IV32-36) yields soft and super stearines, IV 40-42 and 17-21 respectively (Tirtiaux 1998).

A discussion of the fractionation process is beyond the scope of this paper. The reader is referred to a number of reviews (Krishnamurthy and Kellens 1996, Timms 1997, Deffense 1995) covering both the theoretical and practical aspects of fractionation technology.

Zero *trans* margarine fats can be prepared via random interesterification of soybean oil with palm stearine or fully hydrogenated soybean oil in ratios of 80:20 and they concluded that increasing the amount of fully hydrogenated soy to 30 parts produced zero *trans* oils suitable for shortening. 40 parts palm stearine randomized with 60 parts soybean oil also produced shortening oil very similar to commercial products (Petrauskaite *et al*. 1998).

Ozay *et al*. (1996) described the formulation of *trans* free margarines prepared from sunflower and cottonseed oils interesterified with palm oil, palm kernal oil, palm stearine and palm kernal olein and compared them to products made by simply blending the components in various ratios. Palm oil crystallizes slowly compared to other fats and oils leading to a phenomenon known as post hardening in which products become harder upon storage. The authors observed minimal post hardening in their study and reported that the use of skim in preparing the emulsions prior to crystallization was effective in retarding post hardening in blends high in palm and palm kernal oil.

Yusoff *et al*. 1996 reported formulation of *trans* free tub, pastry and bakery margarines from palm oil, palm olein, palm stearine, palm kernal olein interesterified with soybean and rapeseed oil. The normal level of palm oil in commercial soft tub products was reported to be 25% but palm olein can be used up to a level of 40%.

Studies on the use of palm olein in milk fat blends as baking shortenings have been reported (Noraini *et al*. 1998). Blends consisting of 80% palm olein, 60% palm olein and 40% palm olein with hard milk fat fraction and processed in a pilot plant. Baking and sensory tests were compared against a commercial shortening. Noraini *et al*. (1989) studied shortenings formulated from hydrogenated palm oil and palm sterine blended with liquid oils, blends of palm stearine with liquid oils and interesterified (100%) palm oil. They concluded that high palmitic acid oils is best for aeration of fat sugar mixtures but there is no direct relationship between creaming and baking performance. Palm stearine blended with cottonseed oil in a 3:2 ratio produced shortening best suited for aerated fillings. Palm stearine (IV 44) and low eurucic acid rapeseed (11:1) is best in cake baking. For applications in both cream fillings and baking, interesterified palm is the most suitable.

Berger 1998 reported studies on palm oil usage in food products including margarine, vanaspati (a food oil product used extensively in India and Pakistan), baking shortenings, frying fats and dairy products, i.e. whipped toppings, ice cream and cheese. Vanaspati, a butter-like product (melting point 37-38°C) is manufactured with a granular structure and a minimum of free oil at room temperatures. In the early 1980s the product (1,000,000 tons/year), produced in Pakistan from hydrogenated components, contained about 30% *trans* acids. After reformulation with 80% palm oil and 20% liquid vegetable oil, *trans* acids were reduced to less than 4%. However, the saturated acid content would be of the order of 40%.

Analysis of frying oils prepared from rapeseed, sunflower, soybean, peanut and olive blended with 30% palm olein (iodine value minimum 56) show improvement over the 100% liquid oils. Analytical tests (including rancimat at 100 °C, cloud point, free fatty acids, viscosity, polymers, oxidized acids, color and smoke point) were made after 3 days of use. Since extended shelf life is an important consideration in packaged snack foods, the improved oxidative stability of palm oil containing blends has prompted use in Europe and Asia for preparation of instant and fried noodles (Berger 1998).

Oils With Modified Composition

Over the past several decades a number of oilseeds with modified fatty acid compositions have been developed and commercialized. Most have resulted from traditional plant breeding techniques (Lui 1999, Gunstone 2001, Loh 2000, Wilson 1999). These include high and mid-level oleic sunflower oil, high oleic corn, soybean and safflower oil, low linolenic canola and soybeans oils and high oleic/low linolenic canola oil. A number of laboratory frying studies have demonstrated superiority ever commodity oils (Warner and Gupta 2003, Warner and Knowlton 1997, Warner *et al.* 1997, Mounts *et al.* 1994, Warner and Mounts 1993, Su *et al.* 2003). A frying study comparing low linolenic soybean, hydrogenated low linolenic soybean, and high low oleic sunflower against liquid, opaque and heavy duty oils formulated with hydrogenated soybean oils showed that the former group compared well in both fry life and flavor evaluations. Other tests showed that high oleic sunflower and low linolenic soybean oils compare well to hydrogenated oils in spray oil applications and non-dairy creamer formulations. Other applications include fluid margarines/spreads and dressings (Erickson and Frey 1994). Although low linolenic canola and soybeans oils have reached commercialization, costs and production problems have impeded their success in the marketplace (Krawczyk 1999). However, the new labeling regulations may provide new markets and demands for modified composition oils.

The A90, A6 and HS-1 developed by Pioneer, Iowa State University and Hartz Seed Company respectively represent the high saturate soybean oils in which the normal 15% saturated acids have been elevated to as high as 40%. In their natural states these oils lack sufficient solids at temperatures required of a margarine/spread oil. Addition of harder components such as palm oil, interesterified palm oil or cottonseed/soybean stearines shows potential in soft margarine applications (List *et al.* 1996). Owing to the symmetrical nature of their triglyceride structures, the high saturate lines are low, sharply melting materials that, upon random interesterification, melt over a wide range rendering them more amenable to utilization in soft margarine formulation (Kok *et al.* 1999, List *et al.* 1997, List *et al.* 2001). Typically, soft margarines formulated from hydrogenated and liquid soybean oils contain about 10% *trans* fatty acids and about 20% saturated acids. Studies have shown that approximately 25-30% saturated acids are required to formulate zero *trans* soft margarine oils from soybean oil based components (Kok *et al.* 1999, List *et al.* 1995a, List 2001 *et al.*). Thus, any reduction in the *trans* fatty acids will be achieved at the expense of increased saturated acids.

Fluid Shortenings

Fluid shortenings are stable suspensions of 2-20% hard fat in liquid vegetable oil which may or not be hydrogenated (Herzing 1996, Andre and Going 1957, Holman and Quimby 1950, Mitchell 1950). Fluid shortenings have been used in the baking industry for many years where high solids are not required such as fillings, cakes and breads. They serve the same function as solid shortenings by imparting tenderness and lubricity as well as serving as carrier for emulsifiers needed for aerating cake batter of giving crumb strength to bread. Other advantages include the fact that, since they are liquid and pumpable, they can be easily metered into batch and continuous processes. Some reduction of *trans* acids might be achieved by substituting liquid or hydrogenated oil in formulations where hydrogenated oils have been traditionally used.

High Stability Oils

High Stability Oils (HSO) were developed over 30 years ago (Gooding 1972). Compared to commodity oils they are expensive, extremely stable, yet fill definite needs for the food industry. They are liquids at ambient temperature and perform well as spray oils and in applications in products with large surface areas and or where long shelf life is required.

HSO are at least four times more resistant to oxidation and hydrolysis than commodity salad oils which translates in to slower development of off-flavors and color stability shows marked improvements. Typical applications include roasting of nuts, carriers of flavors, use as moisture barriers, as viscosity modifiers, glass enhancers, lubricating/releasing agents, anti-dusting agents and frying operations. The market for HSO use is estimated at 45-57 thousand metric tons in the year 2000 with a breakdown as 70% low-end HSO, 10% mid-range and 20% high-end. These designations refer to their relative stability under active oxygen method conditions (100°C) or hours to reach a peroxide value of 100. Low, mid-range and high-end oils have values of 50-100, 100-300 and >300 respectively (Lampert 2000).

HSO can be processed from both commodity and genetically/plant breeding modified oils. High oleic corn, soybean and sunflower oils meet requirements for low-end HSO without processing beyond refining, bleaching and deodorizing, whereas soybean oil requires partial hydrogenation and dry fractionation as well. Both medium and high-end HSO can be prepared from both commodity and genetically/structurally modified oils. However, light, partial or heavy hydrogenation and dry fractionation must be employed along with the usual refining, bleaching and deodorization steps.

Low-end HSO prepared from hydrogenated, dry fractionated soybean oil contains 15% saturates and 32% *trans*, whereas high oleic sunflower contains 9.5% saturates and 1% *trans*. Canola and high oleic canola based HSO offer opportunity for *trans* reduction in mid-range applications compared to soybean oil. Canola HSO shows *trans* values of 18-29% compared to 51% for soy based oil. Similarly, high oleic based, high-end oils have 33% *trans* compared to 48% for cottonseed/soybean based oils (Lampert 2000).

HSOs are liquids at ambient temperature, highly functional and convenient to use. They are used at low levels often between 0.2 and 1% and are most commonly sprayed onto the surface of the food or ingredient. Although more expensive than commodity oils, processing costs are reduced making final pricing comparable.

It is expected that increased use of HSOs will occur in the future to achieve fat reduction in foods, to improve shelf life and to improve health and nutrition.

Trans **Reduction by Modified Hydrogenation**

A recent report suggests that existing limitations on current equipment is a major obstacle limiting the production of low *trans* oils via hydrogenation (Beers and Mangus 2004a). They indicate that pressures of 50-60 bar (735-882 psi) are needed, while most existing equipment can handle pressures only up to 5 bars (73.5 psi) Hydrogenation at very high pressure, 500-1000 psi (34-60 bars), have been shown to be disadvantageous because significant amounts of high melting triglycerides are formed under these conditions which produce high, flat solid fat index curves (List *et al.* 2000). The insolubility of these highly saturated triglycerides in soybean or other liquid oils render them unsuitable in spreads and of limited use in baking shortening formulations. Most likely, such fats might find use in frying operations (King *et al.* 2001). More recent studies conducted in the author's laboratory have shown, at hydrogenation temperature ranging from 140-170°C and at pressure of 13.6 bar (200 psi), the *trans* fatty acid content can be reduced significantly. At an iodine value of 65 about 17% TFA are produced compared to nearly 40% in commercial hydrogenation. Blending of the IV 65 oil with 70% liquid oil results in spread oils meeting FDA requirements for TFA labeling in the U.S. (Eller *et al.* 2004). Refitting commercial hydrogenation connectors to handle 200 psi pressures should not be difficult.

Over the past decade, catalyst manufacturers have studied *trans* reduction In edible oils (Hasman 1995, Berben *et al.* 1994, Ariaansz and Okonek 1998, Beers and Mangus 2004a, Beers *et al.* 2004b) using both conventional nickel and noble metals such as platinum, palladium and ruthenium. Platinum modified/ammonia catalysts show promise in both TFA reduction and minimization of saturated acids (Berben *et al.* 1994). The use of noble metal catalysts may be limited by cost. Hasman (1995) showed that significant *trans* reduction can be obtained with both canola and soybean oils. However, the rather high catalyst levels required may discourage commercial acceptance along with pressure limitations on equipment.

Several other technologies offer possibilities to reduce TFA during hydrogenation. Harrod and Moller (1999, 2001) and King *et al.* (2001) have reported that hydrogenation in critical fluids such as propane and carbon dioxide produces oils with lowered TFA content. Electrochemical hydrogenation also shows promise for TFA reduction (Warner *et al.* 2000).

About a decade ago it was estimated that about 90% of the world's edible oils were processed by hydrogenation with the remainder by interesterification, fractionation or a combination thereof (Hauman 1994). Recent TFA labeling requirements in the U.S. most likely will result in increased use of alternatives to hydrogenation or modifications of existing hydrogenation methods (Hunter 2004). Since about the year 1998 a number of low/zero *trans* shortenings and spreads have appeared in U.S. markets. Some have been produced by random chemical interesterification of canola oil and fully hydrogenated soybean oil. Others have been produced by enzymatic interesterification of soybean and cottonseed oils. At least one line of products has been produced by modified hydrogenation technology. A number of functional cholesterol lowering spreads have been introduced based on hydrogenation or simple blending of liquid vegetable oils with tropical fats (List 2004b). Thus, it would appear that hydrogenation will continue to be a prominent oil processing technology.

Reformulation for Reduced TFA Content

As discussed in the introduction, reformulation of food products for nutrition labeling presents a number of challenges of both a technical and economic nature. Traditionally, catalytic hydrogenation is the predominant technology of choice. Ideally, reformulation will not increase costs and, in order to meet a zero-gram *trans* fat/serving claim, TFA content must be below 0.5 g. Reformulation must not impair functionality or performance. In order to accomplish this, solid fat and melting points must be maintained. Ideally, replacement of *trans* should not increase saturated acid content. Maintaining oxidative stability and/or shelf life of frying oils and fried foods is an important consideration. Maintaining a consumer friendly label (no hydrogenation) and no cholesterol claim is important, as well as maintaining a major lipid component (i.e. corn, olive) on a label may be important. In addition, maintaining a high level of polyunsaturates (essential, omega 3) is desirable. Last, but not least, it would be desirable to accomplish reformulation with commodity oils or animal fats.

Over the period 1996-2003, soybean oil has averaged slightly over 20 cents/pound, canola 24 cents/pound, cottonseed 25.5 cents/pound and sunflower and corn at about 23 cents/pound. Most of the commodity oils are low in saturated acids (6-15%) with the exception of cottonseed (26%). Lard and beef tallow are cheaper than commodity vegetable oils (15-17% cents/pound) but contain cholesterol and 40-48% saturated acids. Palm oil compares price wise with soybean oil but is high in saturated acids (48%).

Domestic usage of commodity oils over the 1996-2003 period has been dominated by soybean oil, with over 17 billion pounds going into spreads, baking/frying fats and salad/cooking oils. Soybean oil commands over 93% of the spread market, over 88% of the baking/frying market and 73% of the salad/cooking oil market. Traditionally, formulation of soybean oil based products requires hydrogenation for both functionality and oxidative stability as does canola oil.

Applications

The TFA contents of typical food products formulated from hydrogenated soybean oil are given in Table 5.2. The *trans* content of margarines and spreads are taken from the author's laboratory, while the other data comes from technical data sheets supplied by the edible oil processing industry. Soft margarine/spreads and dual purpose salad cooking oils are the lowest in TFA. Stick and hydrogenated clear frying oils are intermediate, while baking and heavy duty frying fats are the highest in TFA content.

Soft margarine (80% fat) requires that the TFA content of the hydrogenated component be slightly less than 5% to meet a zero g/ 14 oz serving claim. Experience has shown that IV 65 soybean oil, produced by hydrogenation under selective conditions, contains about 40% TFA. In order to meet solid fat and melting point requirements for soft margarine (80% fat), about 75% liquid oil is needed, yielding a final TFA content of 10%. Thus, in order to meet the labeling claim, the fat content must be reduced to slightly less than 40%. Such products must be labeled as spreads rather than margarine and may perform poorly in frying and baking. Thus, while reformulation of spreads (less than 80% fat) may be accomplished using traditional hydrogenation methods, soft and stick margarine will require modified methods or other processing techniques such as chemical or enzymatic interesterification, fractionation of tropical oils or trait enhanced oils. Other options include use of multiple processing tools for production of fat blends with the desired physical and functional properties. To date, a number of spreads have been reformulated to meet nutrition labeling requirements for TFA. With the exception of one line of products employing a blend of tropical and unhydrogenated commodity oils, have been reformulated by the aforementioned techniques.

The baking industry employs a number of shortenings whose TFA content varies from 11-25%. Unlike margarine/spreads, these products require higher, flatter solid fat index properties. The industry employs an IV 80 hydrogenated basestock (32-35%) for shortening formulation. Blending with liquid and/or soybean/cottonseed flakes (IV>5%) allows products with varying solid fat profiles required for dif-

TABLE 5.2

Trans TFA and Saturated Acid Content of Hydrogenated Soy Oil Based Food Oils

Food	TFA	g Fat/Serving		
		TFA	Saturated	Saturated + TFA
Soft Margarine	10	1.1	1.6	2.7
Stick Margarine	20	2.2	2.2	4.4
Salad/Frying Oil	10–20	1.0–1.2	2.2–2.5	3.0
Hydro Clear Frying	18	2.5	2.5	5.0
All-Purpose Baking	21	2.9	3.7	6.6
Heavy-Duty Frying	42	5.0	3.0	8.0
Heavy-Duty (Donut Frying)	46	5.5	2.2	7.7

ferent needs. Reformulation of baking shortenings with traditional hydrogenated basestocks will be very difficult. However, it has been reported that hydrogenation of soybean oil with modified nickel catalysts at low temperature and higher pressure yields shortening oils with markedly reduced TFA content meeting the nutrition labeling requirements.

A zero-*trans*, low saturate, all purpose shortening has reached the retail market and has been formulated from liquid sunflower and soybean oils with fully hydrogenated cottonseed oil serving as the hardstock (Scavone 1995). Prior to reformulation, the shortening contained 3.0 g of saturates and 1.9 g of *trans* compared to 2.1 and 0.08 g respectively. Heavy duty and donut-frying shortenings are the highest in TFA content. Not only must they resist oxidation at high temperatures, these fats must contain solids in order to assure that icings and sugars perform on the donuts as intended. Obviously, reformulation of these products for TFA reduction will be extremely difficult.

References

Andre, J. R. and L. H. Going. (1957) Liquid shortening. U.S. Patent 2,815,286.

Anon. (2002) Institute of Medicine of the National Academies of Science, Report on dietary reference intakes for energy, carbohydrates, fiber, fat, fatty acids, cholesterol, protein and amino acids. Chapter 8, pp. 1-99, National Academies Press, Washington, D.C.

Anon. (2003) Food labeling: *Trans* fatty acids in nutrition labeling, final rule. Federal Register. **68** 41433-41506.

Anon. (2004a) United Soy Board, Proposal to Codex Committee on Fats and Oils, Standards for low linolenic and mid oleic soybean oil. Letter to Charles Cooper, FDA Center for Food Safety and Nutrition, College Park, MD.

Anon. (2004b) ADM chooses a trouble-free process for *trans* free fats. Oil Mill Gazetteer. 109 2-5.

Anon. (2005) USDA guidelines for Americans 2005. www.health.gov/dietaryguidelines/dga/document.

Ariaansz, R. F. and D. V. Okonek. (1998) *Trans* isomer control during edible oil processing. In Proceedings of World Conference on Oilseed Processing, Vol. 1. Ed: S. Koseglu, K. Rhee and R. F. Wilson, AOCS Press, Champaign, IL. pp. 77-91.

Beers, A. and G. Mangus. (2004a) Hydrogenation of edible oils for reduced *trans* fatty acid content. Inform. **15**(7) 404-405.

Beers, A., P. Berben, C. Groen, R. Jaqta, G. Lazar, and G. Mangus. (2004b) Lowering the *trans* content of edible oils. Englehard Technical Bulletin, Englehard Corporation, Beachwood, OH. pp. 1-29. Paper presented at 3rd Euro. Fed. Lipid Congress, Edinburgh, Scotland.

Berben, P. H., F. Borninkhof, B. H. Recsink and E. Kuijpers. (1994) Production of low *trans* isomer containing products by hydrogenation. Abstact, American Oil Chemists' Society Meeting, Atlanta, GA. Paper available from Englehard Industries, Beachwood, OH.

Berger, K. (1998) Recent results on palm oil uses in food products. Proceedings of World Conference on Oilseed and Edible Oil Processing, vol. 1. American Oil Chemists' Society, AOCS Press, Champaign, IL. pp. 151-155.

Deffense, E. (1985) Fractionation of Palm Oils. J. Am. Oil. Chem. Soc. **62** 376-385.

Eller, F. J. *et al.* (2004) Submitted to Agricultural and Food Chemistry.

Erickson, N. D. and N. Frey. (1994) Property enhanced oils in food applications. Food Technol. **48** 63-68.

Gillies, M. T. (1974) Shortenings, margarines and food oils. Noyes Data Corporation, Park Ridge, New Jersey. pp. 142-226.

Gooding, C. M. (1972) Production of high stability liquid vegetable oils. U.S. Patent 3,674,821.

Gunstone, F. D. (2001) Oilseed crops with modified fatty acid composition. J. Oleo. Sci. **50** 269-279.

Harrod, M. and P. Moller. (1999) Hydrogenation of substrate and products manufactured according to the process. U.S. Patent 5,962,711.

Harrod, M. and P. Moller. (2001) Partially hydrogenated fatty substances with a low content of *trans* fatty acids. U.S. Patent 6,265,596.

Hasman, J. (1995) *Trans* Suppression in Hydrogenated Oils. Inform **6** 1206-1213.

Haumann, B. F. (1994) Tools: Hydrogenation, interesterification. Inform **5** 668-678.

Herzing, A. C. (1996) Fluid shortenings in bakery products. Inform. **7** 165-167.

Holman, G. W. and O. T. Quimby. (1950) Process of preparing suspensions of solid triglyceride and liquid oil. U.S. Patent 2,521,219.

Hunter, J. E. (2004) Alternatives to *trans* fatty acids in foods. Inform. **15**(8) 510-512.

King, J. W., R, L, Holliday, G. R. List, and J. M. Snyder. (2001) Hydrogenation of soybean oil in supercritical carbon dioxide and hydrogen. J. Am. Oil Chem. Soc. **78** 107-113.

Kok, L. L., W. R. Fehr, E. G. Hammond, and P. J. White. (1999) *Trans* margarine from highly saturated soybean oil. J. Am. Oil. Chem. Soc. **76** 1175-1181.

Krawczyk, T. (1999) Edible specialty oils:An unfulfilled promise. Inform. **10** 555-561.

Krishnamurthy, R. ands M. Kellens. (1996) Fractionation and winterization. In Bailey's Industrial Oil and Fat Products, 5th edition. Ed: Y. H. Hui, John Wiley and Sons, New York. pp. 301-337.

Lampert, D. (2000) High stability oils: What are they? How are they made? and Why do we need them. In Physical Properties of Fats, Oils and emulsifiers. Ed: N. Widlak. American Oil Chemists' Society, AOCS Press, Champaign, IL. pp. 238-246.

List, G. R., E. A. Emken, W. F. Kwolek, T. D. Simpson, and H. J. Dutton. (1977) "Zero *trans*" margarines: Preparation, structure, and properties of interesterified soybean oil-soy trisaturate blends. J. Am. Oil Chem. Soc. **54** 408-413.

List, G. R., T. Pelloso, F. Orthoefer, M. Chrysam, and T. L. Mounts. (1995a) Preparation and properties of zero *trans* soybean oil margarines, J. Am. Oil Chem. Soc. **72** 383-384.

List, G. R., T.L. Mounts, F. Orthoefer, and W. E. Neff. (1995b) Margarine and shortening oils by interesterification of liquid and trisaturated triglycerides. J. Am. Oil Chem. Soc. **72** 379-382.

List, G. R., T. L. Mounts, F. Orthoefer and W. E. Neff. (1996) Potential margarine oils from genetically modified soybeans. J. Am. Oil Chem. Soc. **73** 729-732.

List, G. R., T.L. Mounts, F. Orthoefer, and W. E. Neff. (1997) Effect of interesterification on the structure and physical properties of high stearic acid soybean oils. J. Am. Oil Chem. Soc. **74** 327-329.

List, G.R., Neff, W.E., Holliday, R.L., King, J.W., and Holzer, R. (2000) Hydrogenation of soybean oil triglycerides: Effect of pressure on selectivity. J. Am. Oil Chem. Soc. 77:311-314.

List, G. R., T. Pelloso, F. Orthoefer, K. Warner, and W. E. Neff. (2001) Soft margarines from high stearic acid soybean oils. J. Am. Oil. Chem. Soc. **78** 103-104.

List, G. R. (2004a) Decreasing *trans* and saturated fatty acid content in food oils. Food Technol. **58**(1) 23-31.

List, G. R. (2004b) Processing and reformulation for nutrition labeling of *trans* fatty acids. Lipid Technol. **16**(8) 173-177.

Loh, W. (2000) Biotechnology and vegetable oils: First generation products in the marketplace. In Physical Properties of Fats, Oils and emulsifiers. Ed: N. Widlak. American Oil Chemists' Society, AOCS Press, Champaign, IL. pp. 247-253.

Lui, K. (1999) Soy oil modifications: Products and applications. Inform **10** 868-877.

Mitchell, P. J. (1950) Permanently pumpable oleaginous suspensions. U.S. Patent 2,521,242.

Mounts, T. L., K. Warner, G. R. List, W. E. Neff and R. F. Wilson. (1994) Low linolenic acid soybean oil—alternatives to frying oils. J. Am. Oil Chem. Soc. **71** 495-499.

Noraini, I., K. Berger and S. Hong. (1989) Evaluation of shortenings based on various palm oil products. J. Am. Oil Chem. Soc. **46** 481-493.

Noraini, I., C. Chemaimon and H. Hanriah. (1998) The use of palm olein: Hard milk fat blends as baking shortenings. Proceedings of World Conference on Oilseed and Edible Oil Processing, vol. 1. American Oil Chemists' Society, AOCS Press, Champaign, IL. pp. 147-155.

Ozay, G., M. Yildiz, M. Mahidin, M. Yusoff, M. Yurdagul and N. Goken (1998) Proceedings of World Conference on Oilseed and Edible Oil Processing, vol. 1. American Oil Chemists' Society, AOCS Press, Champaign, IL. pp. 143-146.

Petrauskaite, V. W., DeGreyt, M. Kellens and A. Huyghaebaert. (1998) Physical and chemical properties of *trans* free fats produced by chemical interesterification of vegetable oil blends. J. Am. Oil Chem. Soc. **75** 489-493.

Rozendall, A. and A. R. Macrae. (1997) Interesterification of oils and fats. In Lipid Technologies and Applications. Ed: F. Gunstone, Marcel Dekker, New York. pp. 223-263.

Su, C., M. Gupta, and P. White. (2003) Oxidative and flavor stabilities of soybean oils with low and ultra-low linolenic acid composition. J. Am. Oil Chem. Soc. **80** 171-176.

Scavone, T. A. (1995) Beta prime stable, low saturate, low *trans*, all purpose shortening. U.S. Patent 5,470,598.

Timms, R.E. (1997) Fractionation. In: F. Gunstone (ed.), Lipid Technologies and Applications, Marcel Dekker, New York. pp. 199-222.

Tirtiaux, A. (1998) Dry fractionation – The beat goes on. Proceedings World Conference on Oilseed Processing. AOCS Press, Champaign, IL. pp. 92-98.

Warner, K. and S. Knowlton. (1997) Frying oils and oxidative stability of high-oleic corn oils. J. Am. Oil Chem. Soc. **74** 1317-1322.

Warner, K. and T. L. Mounts. (1993) Frying stability of soybean and canola oils with modified fatty acid compositions. J. Am. Oil Chem. Soc. **70** 983-988.

Warner, K., P. Orr, and M. Glynn. (1997) Effect of fatty acid composition of oils on flavor and stability of fried foods. J. Am. Oil Chem. Soc. **74** 347-356.

Warner, K., W. E. Neff, G. R. List and P. Pintauro. (2000) Electrochemical hydrogenation of edible oils in a solid polymer electrolyte reactor. Sensory and compositional characteristics of low *trans* oils. J. Am. Oil Chem. Soc. **77** 1113-1117.

Warner, K. and M. Gupta. (2003) Frying quality and stability of ultra low and low linolenic acid soybean oils. J. Am. Oil Chem. Soc. **80** 275-280.

Wilson, R. F. (1999) Alternatives to genetically modified soybeans – The better bean initiative. Lipid Technol. **11** 107-109.

Yusoff, M., H. Kifli, H. Noorlida, and M. P. Rozig. (1998) Formulation of *trans*-free margarines. In Proceedings of World Conference on Oilseed Processing, vol. 1. Ed: S. Koseglu, K. Rhee and R. F. Wilste, AOCS Press, Champaign, IL. pp. 156-158.

Chapter 6

Communicating with Consumers About *trans* Fat: The Importance of Consumer Research

Shelley Goldberg, Susan T. Borra, and Diane Quagliani

International Food Information Council, 1100 Connecticut Ave, NW, Ste 430, Washington DC 20036; goldberg@ific.org

Introduction

In recent years, media coverage about the link between *trans* fat and cardiovascular health has increased (ANON, 2004a) and, in preparation for the FDA requirement that the *trans* fat content of packaged foods appear on the Nutrition Facts label by January 1, 2006, many food companies already list this information on food labels. These factors are contributing to a heightened awareness of *trans* fat among consumers.

However, while qualitative research with consumers indicates that they identify *trans* fat as a type of fat to limit, even those identifying themselves as "nutritionally savvy" are unable to specify why some fats are more healthful than others. In fact, consumers generally are overwhelmed and confused about different types of fat (ANON, 2004b). When asked how knowledgeable they consider themselves to be about *trans* fat, 63% of consumers said they consider themselves "not at all knowledgeable" and 22% consider themselves "a little knowledgeable." Only 13% consider themselves "somewhat knowledgeable" and 2% consider themselves "very knowledgeable" about *trans* fat (ANON, 2003b).

One important goal of including information about *trans* fat on the Nutrition Facts label is to help consumers choose a more healthful diet. Yet, consumers may not interpret or apply information on the food label as intended, as indicated by research that investigated consumers' understanding of a proposed food label footnote on *trans* fat.

Testing Consumer Understanding of a *trans* Fat Footnote on the Nutrition Facts Label

In addition to FDA's rule to include *trans* fat on the Nutrition Facts label of food packages as a separate line item, the agency explored including a footnote to explain *trans* fat in the context of the diet. The proposed footnote read, "Intake of *trans* fat should be as low as possible" (ANON, 2004a). This statement was based upon the Institute of Medicine's 2002 report on dietary reference intakes for macronutrients, which did not provide quantitative dietary guidance for *trans* fat, but instead recommended that intake of *trans* fat be as low as possible while consuming a nutritionally adequate diet (ANON, 2002b).

To measure consumer interpretation and use of a Nutrition Facts label that included the proposed *trans* fat footnote, the International Food Information Council (IFIC) Foundation commissioned quantitative research (ANON, 2003b).

The research sample consisted of 1,301 primary household shoppers ages 18 and older and was weighted to be representative of the U.S. population. The survey was administered via the Internet so consumers could compare pairs of Nutrition Facts labels and identify the healthier choice between related unbranded products containing similar amounts of calories and total fat.

Consumers were exposed to three pairs of Nutrition Facts labels. The first pair reflected the current state of nutrition labels (no *trans* fat listed). The second pair included quantitative information for *trans* fat (grams of fat per serving). The third pair featured both quantitative information for *trans* fat and the FDA proposed *trans* fat footnote. Each respondent was shown a single type of food: an entrée, a frozen dinner, microwave popcorn, chips or a spread (butter versus margarine). The labels used for spreads are shown in Figure 6.1.

Consumers Give trans Fat Footnote Too Much Weight

Results showed that across a variety of food products labeled with the *trans* fat footnote, the vast majority of consumers repeatedly identified the product without *trans* fat as the healthier choice, based upon aided awareness of the footnote.

In the case of spreads and frozen dinners, when consumers were shown labels containing the *trans* fat footnote and asked to identify the healthier product, the majority of consumers chose the product without *trans* fat, even when the amount of *trans* fat and saturated fat combined was less than the saturated fat in the *trans* fat-free product.

Specifically, in the case of spreads (butter vs. margarine), consumers overwhelmingly chose butter (with 7 grams of saturated fat and 0 grams of *trans* fat) over margarine (2 grams of saturated fat and 2 grams of *trans* fat) as the healthier choice. In contrast, when shown these products with the current label (no *trans* fat information), most selected margarine as the healthier choice. When shown these products with only *trans* fat quantitative data appearing on the label (i.e., without the footnote) butter and margarine were selected as the healthier choice about equally as often. Figure 6.2 illustrates these findings.

Figure 6.3 summarizes consumers' selections of the healthier choice across all five product categories. In each product category, there was an inverse relationship between the amount of *trans* fat information provided on the Nutrition Facts label and the percentage of consumers choosing the product with no *trans* fat as the healthier choice.

When consumers used the current Nutrition Facts label to ascertain a product's overall healthfulness, they tended to rely on a variety of components such as calories, total fat, sodium and saturated fat. When the *trans* fat line item was added, consumers were able to use that information, in addition to the other components, to make their choice. Therefore, the addition of a separate line item for *trans* fat appears to be a use-

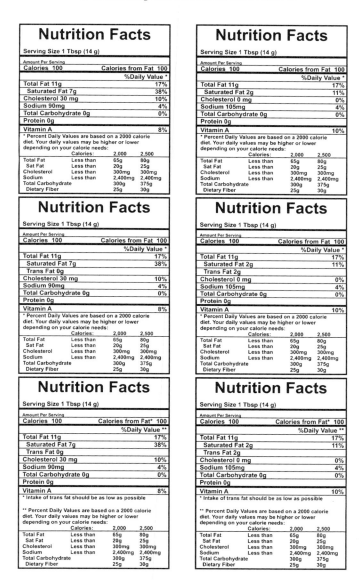

Fig. 6.1. Consumers were asked to compare pairs of Nutrition Facts labels and identify the healthier choice between similar unbranded products containing similar amounts of calories and total fat. The labels displayed varying amounts of information about *trans* fat.

ful tool for consumers. However, when consumers used the Nutrition Facts label containing the proposed *trans* fat footnote, they placed disproportionate weight on the *trans* fat nutrition information, discounting other important content information.

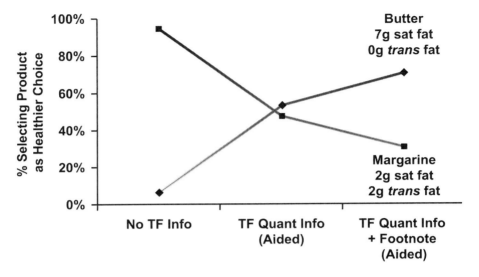

Fig. 6.2. When shown labels for spreads containing a *trans* fat footnote, most consumers chose the product without *trans* fat as the healthier choice, even when the amount of *trans* fat and saturated fat combined in the product was less than the saturated fat in the product without *trans* fat.

When consumers were asked why they chose the product without *trans* fat as the healthier choice when the footnote was present, they almost always cited the *trans* fat content, overlooking information about calories, total fat, sodium, saturated fat, cholesterol or other components. They tended to say the footnote conveyed that *trans* fat is very unhealthy and should be avoided. In fact, when consumers were asked about the healthfulness of *trans* fat relative to saturated fat based upon the footnote, nearly eight out of 10 (78%) respondents agreed with the statement, "*Trans* fat is worse for you than saturated fat."

Points to Consider for Successful Communication

These research findings indicate that when it comes to nutrition information, consumers do not always receive the intended message.

In this research, consumers' misinterpretation of the "healthfulness" of products based on the proposed *trans* fat footnote underscores the importance of conducting consumer research to develop effective public health messages. Communicators and educators can obtain a wealth of feedback from consumers through formal research techniques such as focus groups, in-home observations and quantitative surveys. But informal channels also provide valuable insights. For example, health professionals can test messages about *trans* fat with patients, clients, friends, family or coworkers who resemble the intended audience.

		Spread		Frozen Dinner		Popcorn		Chips		Entree	
		A	B	A	B	A	B	A	B	A	B
Total Fat:		11g	11g	35g	35g	9g	11g	8g	8g	37g	35g
Saturated Fat:		7g	2g	18g	9g	4.5g	1.5g	2.5g	1.5g	15g	11g
Trans Fat		0g	2g	0g	5g	0g	3g	0g	3.5g	0g	8g
Current Label Format with No *Trans* Fat Information		6%	94%	5%	95%	63%	37%	3%	97%	6%	94%
Quantitative Information on *Trans* Fat (Aided)		53%	47%	60%	40%	83%	17%	66%	34%	60%	40%
Quantitative Information + Footnote (Aided)		70%	30%	82%	18%	96%	4%	79%	21%	80%	20%

Fig. 6.3. Addition of a footnote about *trans* fat to the Nutrition Facts label resulted in most consumers selecting a product with no *trans* fat as the healthier choice regardless of saturated fat content.

To help consumers better understand dietary fat, communicators should use clear and simple language to discuss the different types of dietary fats and to define terms such as *trans* fat, saturated fat and cholesterol. Rather than providing consumers with general advice such as "keep *trans* fat intake as low as possible," offer specific information on which foods contain *trans* fat and small, easy-to-implement steps for decreasing *trans* fat intake. Instead of using a "one-size-fits-all" communications approach, provide personalized tips that suit consumers' particular lifestyle challenges. Most important, put *trans* fat into perspective so consumers don't focus attention on one nutrient at the expense of an overall balanced diet.

Research indicates that consumers feel overwhelmed by what they perceive as a bombardment of confusing and contradictory nutrition messages and, so, are tuning out these messages (ANON, 2002c). Technological advances such as the Internet increase consumer access to health information, but also seem to decrease their ability to identify credible sources of information.

To clear up consumer confusion, it's vital that health communicators across all disciplines "speak with one voice" about *trans* fat and other dietary guidance to the largest possible audience. An important way to achieve this goal is for parties that communicate with consumers—including the government, health professional organizations, the food industry, academia, the media and nutrition educators—to partner together on their communications to send consumers clear and consistent nutrition messages. Individual health communicators also play an important role by conveying consistent information during individual counseling and other educational contacts with consumers. The following section includes answers to common consumer questions about *trans* fat to assist communicators with consumer messaging about *trans* fat.

Answers to Common Consumer Questions about *trans* Fat

What are trans *fats?*

Trans fats are unsaturated fatty acids formed when vegetable oils are processed and made more solid or into a more stable liquid. This processing is called hydrogenation. *Trans* fats also occur naturally in low amounts in some foods including, milk, cheese, and animal fats.

Trans fats from all sources provide two to four percent of total calories compared with 12 percent from saturated fat and 34 percent from total fat in the American diet. The majority of *trans* fats come from processed foods. About one-fifth of the *trans* fats in the diet come from animal sources such as certain meats and dairy products.

What foods contain trans *fats?*

Trans fats are present in variable amounts in a wide range of foods, including most foods made with partially hydrogenated oils, such as baked goods and fried foods, and some margarine products. *Trans* fats also occur naturally in low amounts in certain meats and dairy products.

Why are trans *fats in foods?*

Trans fats form when an oil is partially hydrogenated. The process converts oils into a more stable liquid or semi-solid form.

Partially hydrogenated oils are used in processed foods because they help produce high quality food products that stay fresh longer and have a more desirable texture. It is not always possible to substitute unhydrogenated oils because of differences in the way the oils work to produce acceptable food products.

For example, by using partially hydrogenated vegetable oil to make some margarine products, manufacturers can produce a spreadable topping that is lower in saturated fat than butter and can be used immediately upon removal from the refrigerator. Likewise, manufacturers can produce shortenings to make French fries, flaky piecrusts and crispy crackers. Products made with partially hydrogenated oils also resist rancidity (when fats develop an "off" flavor) longer than those using unhydrogenated oils. Foods that contain these oils must list "partially hydrogenated vegetable oil" in the ingredient statement of the food label.

Are partially hydrogenated oils used for any other reasons?

Fats and oils containing *trans* fats are used in place of baking and frying fats that have higher levels of saturated fats. Examples of fats with higher levels of saturated fats include lard, butter and highly saturated vegetable oils like palm, palm kernel and coconut oils. In the mid-1980s, the food industry responded to recommendations from health authorities and interest from consumers to reduce the amount of highly saturated vegetable oils along with animal fats in the food supply. The best, and in many cases the only, available alternative was to reformulate products by substituting partially hydrogenated vegetable oils for the highly saturated fats.

How do trans fats, saturated fats and dietary cholesterol impact blood cholesterol?

The National Academy of Sciences' Institute of Medicine (IOM) (ANON, 2002b) concluded that saturated fat, *trans* fat and dietary cholesterol all raise blood LDL cholesterol (the "bad" cholesterol). In addition, some evidence suggests that intake of *trans* fats lowers HDL cholesterol (the "good" cholesterol).

How does blood cholesterol relate to heart disease?

High blood cholesterol is one risk factor for cardiovascular heart disease. People with high blood cholesterol levels are more likely to develop the disease.

What other factors play a role in heart disease?

Cardiovascular disease is very complex. While blood fats such as cholesterol play a part in the development of the disease, there are a number of other factors involved such as diabetes, hypertension, blood clotting, gender, age and heredity.

In addition, lifestyle factors other than diet play key roles in the development of heart disease. Research clearly shows that increased physical activity and maintaining a healthy weight are critical factors in reducing risk for cardiovascular disease.

Should I reduce my intake of trans fat?

The IOM recommended that the intake of *trans* fat as well as saturated fat and cholesterol should be as low as possible while consuming a nutritionally adequate diet. Because *trans* fat, saturated fat, and cholesterol are difficult to avoid in ordinary, non-vegan diets, consuming none would require significant changes to the total diet. According to the IOM, such changes may have undesirable effects, which may result in inadequate intakes of protein and certain micronutrients. More research is needed to determine realistic levels of *trans* and saturated fat and cholesterol intakes that are consistent with a nutritionally adequate diet for different population groups.

The contribution of saturated fat to American diets is much greater than that of *trans* fat. Individuals in the United States consume five to six times the level of saturated fats than *trans* fat.

How can I reduce the amount of trans *fat in my diet?*

- You can lower the amount of *trans* fat in your diet by following the advice of health professionals:
- Reducing total fat intake generally will help lower your intake of saturated fat, *trans* fat and cholesterol.
- Reducing *trans* fat intake should not be accomplished by substituting food higher in saturated fat in the diet.
- Monounsaturated and polyunsaturated fats may be substituted while keeping total fat intake moderate.

What food choices can I make to help lower intake of saturated fat and trans *fat in my diet?*

Most liquid vegetable oils are naturally lower in saturated fat and are *trans* fat-free. These include soybean, canola, corn, olive, safflower and sunflower oils.

Margarine products contain significantly lower amounts of saturated fat than animal fats such as butter, tallow, and lard, or solid shortenings. And, many margarine products are low in *trans* fat or are *trans* fat-free. (Remember that liquid and lower fat versions of margarines do not substitute well in recipes where shortening, stick margarine or butter is required.)

New fat processing technologies have produced some *trans* fat-free products. Additional products will likely become available in the near future.

To lower intake of saturated fat and *trans* fat, try reduced-fat, low-fat, fat-free and *trans* fat-free versions of frequently consumed foods.

Is trans *fat included on the Nutrition Facts label?*

The FDA regulates what is put on the Nutrition Facts label of most processed foods. (The USDA regulates labeling for meats, fish and poultry products.)

The FDA published the final rule for *trans* fat labeling on July 9, 2003. The new label will require a *trans* fat line to be declared directly under the saturated fat line of the Nutrition Facts panel on all products with a measurable level of *trans* fat (at least 0.5 grams per serving). This rule will be effective January 1, 2006; however, food and beverage companies are allowed to add the *trans* fat line before the deadline.

FDA currently requires that total fat, saturated fat and cholesterol be listed on the Nutrition Facts panel. This requirement grew out of years of scientific research and dietary recommendations by major health and nutrition organizations. Currently, the Daily Values for total fat, saturated fat and cholesterol are based on the science available at the time of the implementation of the Nutrition Labeling and Education Act (NLEA) of 1990. The NLEA requires that nutrients listed in the Nutrition Facts panel be declared in a manner that helps consumers understand the contribution of a food to the total daily intake of that nutrient. The % Daily Value has been added to food labels for this purpose.

The recommendations of the IOM suggest that intakes of saturated fat and cholesterol, as well as *trans* fat, be as low as possible while consuming a nutritionally adequate diet.

However, the IOM did not provide sufficient information for FDA to set a Daily Value for *trans* fat. A separate IOM expert committee was convened to identify general guiding principles for using the Dietary Reference Intakes in food labeling and examine the best way to communicate the Institute of Medicine's dietary guidance for *trans* fat, saturated fat, and cholesterol on food labels. FDA received the Committee's report in 2003 and will be responsible for taking the next steps to determine appropriate uses of Dietary Reference Intakes in food labeling.

References

Anon., 2002a. Food & Drug Administration. Food Labeling: *Trans* Fatty Acids in Nutrition Labeling, Nutrient Content Claims, and Health Claims; Reopening of the Comment Period. Food & Drug Administration Web site. 2002. Available at: http://www.fda.gov/OHRMS/DOCKETS/98fr/02-29096.htm.

Anon., 2002b. Institute of Medicine. Dietary Reference Intakes for Energy, Carbohydrate, Fiber, Fat, Fatty Acids, Cholesterol, Protein, and Amino Acids (Macronutrients). The National Academies Press Web site.2002. Available at: http://www.nap.edu/books/0309085373/html/.

Anon., 2002c. International Food Information Council Foundation. How Consumers Feel about Food and Nutrition Messages. International Food Information Council Web site. 2002. Available at: http://www.ific.org/research/newconvres.cfm.

Anon., 2003a. Food Labeling. *Trans* Fatty Acids In Nutrition Labeling, Final Rule Federal Reg. 41433–41506

Anon., 2003c. International Food Information Council Foundation. Questions and Answers About *Trans* Fats. International Food Information Council Web site. 2003. Available at: http://www.ific.org/publications/qa/*trans*qa.cfm.

Anon., 2004a. Center for Media and Public Affairs. Food For Thought V - *Reporting of Diet, Nutrition, and Food Safety News.* International Food Information Council Web site. 2004. Available at: http://www.ific.org/research/fftres.cfm.

Anon., 2004b. International Food Information Council Foundation. Fitting dietary fats into a healthful diet—a consumer point of view. International Food Information Council Web site. 2004. Available at: http://www.ific.org/research/fatsres.cfm.

Chapter 7

Trans Fat Reformulation Is Not a Technical Objective!

Willie Loh

Cargill Specialty Canola Oils, P.O. Box 5693; Minneapolis, MN 55440; Willie_Loh@Cargill.com

Introduction

With the approach of a January 1, 2006 deadline to disclose *trans* fatty acids in processed foods, many food companies are busily engaged to reformulate their products to a "*trans* free" status. They have hired outside consultants, called in their fats and oils suppliers and charged their product development function with eliminating *trans* fat from the Nutrition Fact panel without affecting product functionality, taste and any other product features discernible to the consumer. At this writing, the U.S. Food and Drug Administration (FDA) labeling regulations do not define claims for "*trans* fat free" or "low in *trans* fat." The terms "*trans* free" and "zero *trans*" are used here to mean less than 0.5 gm of *trans* fat per serving. The term "*trans* reformulation" refers to the processes for reducing and/or eliminating *trans* fat content.

A survey of industry efforts since the announcement of these guidelines in July of 2003 suggests *trans* reformulation may be far more difficult than most have envisioned. Some of the reformulation efforts will be scrapped before they reach commercial production because either the technical objectives were unrealistic or the resulting products do not match commercial requirements. In such cases, the reformulated products may reach the marketplace with compromises in both nutritional profile and taste. The product development functions responsible for reformulation will be working feverishly to launch improved versions to follow the initial launch.

There will also be companies with successful reformulated products on the store shelves long before the January 1, 2006 deadline. The consumer will not be able to discern any organoleptic differences in these products. Nevertheless, attention will be drawn to them because their packaging will communicate the nutritional benefits of "zero *trans*." The reformulated products and the nutritional advantages they deliver will be consistent with, and even enhance, the brand positioning.

Many companies focus solely on the regulations published by the FDA dealing with *trans* fat content in processed foods. Regulations, however, can and often do change. Not understanding the social, political and economic forces driving such regulatory action can be short sighted. If regulations change, then additional rounds of production reformulation may be necessary. Each reformulation is not only expensive and each version of the reformulated product runs the risk of deviating from the original and alienating the customer. A more strategic approach involves analyzing the forces driving the marketplace and government regulations and reformulating toward an objective consistent with real trends.

The difference between the successful and unsuccessful efforts to reduce or eliminate *trans* fatty acids will be discussed.

What Are These Trends?

For the past two decades, food companies have been accused of contributing to a litany of health problems. These include increased incidence of high blood pressure, cardiovascular disease, hypertension, stroke, diabetes, metabolic syndrome and obesity related deaths. Media reports have focused on dietary profiles that contribute to these diseases, including high salt, high fat, high saturated fat, high carbohydrates and of course, *trans* fatty acids. In most cases, nutritionists have not established causal relationships between specific dietary profiles and disease development. Even where good correlations exist, genetics and lifestyle choices can significantly alter these relationships. However, nutritional studies do not necessarily drive consumer perception. The average consumer is not a biochemist and is unable to understand the science behind these concerns. Rather, the consumer focuses on a much simpler matter—personal health.

Consumers do not have to be public health experts to be aware of the staggering statistics for growing obesity in the population, the increased incidence of cardiovascular disease or diabetes. Consumers do not need to understand the relationship of metabolic syndrome to developments of diabetes, e.g. blindness, insulin dependency, etc. Consumers do not need to follow the relationship of high LDL-cholesterol levels to cardiovascular disease. They only have to look at all their family members or a small group of closed friends to know that their personal health may be affected by diet.

For a variety of reasons, consumers have blamed the foods they eat as a root cause of the obesity crisis. They expect food companies to provide them with healthier foods. If not, they may switch brands or select other food categories. For example, rocked by criticism of high carbohydrate content and *trans* fat, the consumption of potato products dropped by 5% between the first quarter of 2003 and the first quarter of 2004. Approximately seven billion pounds of potato products are consumed annually in North America. A 5% drop represents a reduction of 350,000,000 pounds of fried potatoes. Everyone in the industry, from the potato grower, to the seed grower, the par fryer, the oil manufacturer, the salt manufacturer, the trucking company, the railroad, the retailers and the food service establishment were impacted by a reduction in total market size.

Therefore, if consumers perceive certain products to be unhealthy, food manufacturers will either have to make substantial improvements or see a potential reduction in market size. Foods that are consumed for lifestyle reasons, e.g. snack foods, risk losing their "share of stomach" if they are perceived to be unhealthy. While such "lifestyle" categories may not have a healthy image, neither are they perceived as harmful. No one wants to eat unhealthy food.

Consumer perception is also driven by activist groups who assume a policing role in public health. The Center for Science in the Public Interest and BanTransFat.com are two organizations that have effectively focused media attention on *trans* fat in the American diet. Media savvy, these relatively small groups have achieved a high consumer profile compared to traditional public health organizations such as the American Heart Association.

Recently, these activist groups have successfully used the courts to create adverse publicity for major brands. They typically attack the strongest brands through a combination of advertising, lawsuits and public relations efforts to generate news stories. Their targets are the iconic brands that have been carefully built through decades of corporate communication. Quality and safety are attributes built into all strong brands. When these brands are in danger, the companies behind them react quickly to limit the damage. Initially, these groups organized class action suits claiming damage to entire segments of society. More recently, they have focused legal action on brands that appeal to children.

Although activist groups have increased consumer awareness of the link between poor nutrition and disease, the requirement for disclosing *trans* fat content in processed foods results from government regulation. The food industry has argued that food ingredients are legal and the over consumption and the lack of exercise contribute more to obesity and diabetes than food products themselves. The federal government, however, has aggressively pursued *trans* fat labeling because of the impact of two major demographic trends: high Medicare costs and retirement of the baby boomer generation.

Despite significant structural shifts to contain medical costs, the bill for Medicare benefits continue to outpace inflation. The cost of Medicare is expected to climb even faster as the baby boomer generation begins to retire in the next five years. One way for the U.S. government to contain Medicare costs is to promote the development of healthier foods. Including *trans* fat in the Nutrition Fact panel is one of the many regulatory changes underway to stimulate the development of healthier food options in the market place. A new class of regulations to permit qualified health claims on food packages is another.

In the first decade of the 21st century, we see the confluence of three developments that are imposing tremendous pressure on food companies to introduce healthier food products: (i) A dramatic increase in obesity and obesity related disease in the population; (ii) Manipulation of the media and the court system by activist groups to create negative publicity for major brands; and (iii) Proliferation of labeling regulations to encourage the development of healthier foods.

When seen in the overarching context of public health, *trans* fat labeling is only one part of a larger effort to control health care costs by guiding consumers to select healthier foods. Since *trans* labeling alone will not solve the problem of obesity and diabetes, additional government regulations to stimulate the development of healthier food options should be anticipated.

How Can Food Companies Respond?

Food companies, like any other type of company, can only satisfy their customers by providing solutions that their customers perceive as valuable. Before beginning a *trans* reformulation effort, food companies have to understand how their consumers perceive the nutritional qualities of their branded products. What do the consumers expect from their brand? If the food manufacturer builds in a feature, e.g. reduced or zero *trans* fat, will the consumer perceive this as an added benefit? If the brand already promises good nutrition, how will consumer perception of the brand be affected by *trans* reduction or *trans* elimination?

The consumer is neither a biochemist nor a food scientist. He does not know what makes certain food products healthier than others. However, the consumer makes purchase decisions everyday among competitive products. Analysis of the consumer's decision making process can determine if nutrition drives purchasing intent and the value placed on improved nutrition, if any.

With nine months left before the labeling regulations goes into effect, the food companies which have successfully completed *trans* reformulation effort are the ones who understand how consumers will react to the *trans* fat status of their brands and established reformulation objectives which are consistent with their brand promise. In effect, the first step in *trans* reformulation is to define the business objective. The technical objectives, i.e. permissible *trans* fat level and ingredient listing, follows establishment of the business objective.

Identifying those features the consumer perceives to be beneficial is absolutely critical to the process. Technical objectives cannot be defined without a clearly articulated brand position. Business objectives, as defined by consumer perception, define the technical approach—not the other way around.

What Can Consumers Tell You?

Consumers do not understand lipid biochemistry. They do not keep track of the technical literature on nutritional studies. American consumers, however, have always trusted government regulation on food products. Whether they understand all the information is unclear. It is unlikely that the amount of various fat types (expressed as grams of fat per serving) means very much, unless that number is zero. The number of consumers that understand the meaning of "% Daily Value" is also unknown. Since the Nutrition Facts panel underwent its last major change in 1985, however, the majority of consumers claim that they review this information before purchasing a food product.

If 50% of the consumers examine the back of packaged food products for nutritional information, including the ingredient statement, then 100% of consumers look at the front of the packaging. Consumer surveys show that nutritional claims on the front, often highlighted in starbursts or colored flags, are read and accepted as valid. Food companies add such front of the package nutritional claims because they can influence purchase intent. The degree to which such nutritional claims create competitive advantages can be readily tested.

Beginning in 2002, long before the *trans* fat labeling guidelines were first proposed, we began to test consumer reaction to potential nutritional claims on the front of the package. Not all the claims were defined then and some are still under consideration. Nevertheless, the test results clearly showed that consumers accept such claims as valid and rely on them to make healthy choices. These tests were conducted on a random sample of U.S. women in the workforce who had access to a computer.

The subjects were contacted by e-mail and invited to respond to a short survey. Participation was voluntary and no payment was made as a result of their participation. The subjects were not made aware of the test objectives and received no prior communication on dietary fats, product labeling or related topics.

The test subjects were shown two pictures: a standard food package, and one with health claims added. Figure 7.1a shows a breakfast cereal. Figure 7.1b showed the same product with some health claims added. (Real brands were used in the actual test.) The test subjects were asked four open-ended questions:

- Do you buy this product?
- Which package do you prefer?
- Why did you choose that one?
- If package A costs X, how much would you pay for package B?

Their unaided responses are summarized in Table 7.1.

As expected, almost all subjects purchased breakfast cereal. If a small percentage of the respondents reported familiarity with the product, then only their responses would be calculated. But because the response was nearly unanimous, there was essentially no difference between the total response and those that purchase breakfast cereals regularly.

Almost all the subjects chose box B over box A, even though nothing in the instructions directed their attention to the health claims. In response to the second question, the overwhelming reason given for choosing box B over box A was health. The choice was made because of the front of the package nutrition claim, even though the test subjects had received no prior information on nutrition. Because they were selected at random, there was no reason to expect that they would have any greater interest or knowledge in nutrition than typical consumers. The results show that consumers associate nutritional claims with improved health.

The answer to the last question was also surprising. A large percentage of consumers expressed a belief that box B delivered more value by suggesting a higher price point. This was also an open-ended question. The price of $3.09 for Box A was the actual retail price for a branded breakfast cereal in the Midwest. The consumers volunteered their own value for box B. The results suggest that consumers are will-

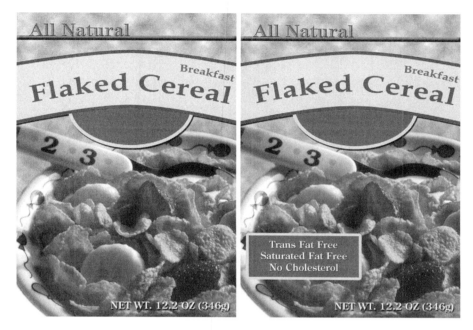

Fig. 7.1. Breakfast cereal with (1a) and without (1b) nutritional claims.

ing to pay more for products that they perceive to deliver specific health benefits.

Using a similar approach, tests were conducted on multiple product categories. While breakfast cereal is perceived to be a "healthy" product category, both "healthy" and "less healthy" products were tested. Within each category, multiple brands were tested. A number of different product claims were tested in different combinations. A few general conclusions are provided.

Regardless of the product category tested, consumers showed strong preference for those products with nutritional claims on the front of the package. Regardless of the consumer perception of a specific product category as delivering "nutrition" or "lifestyle" benefits, consumers always preferred to purchase the healthier version. Not surprisingly, no one wanted to eat unhealthy food.

Within each product category, the leading brands were compared against themselves with or without health claims. The tests consistently showed that the choice of brands had virtually no impact on the consumer response. Whether it was the leading national brand or a private label brand, the percentage of consumers choosing the healthier option was always higher and comparable. The premium that the consumer subjects volunteered to pay was similar within each product category, suggesting that consumers have set values for improved nutrition.

The test results also showed that consumers react to specific nutritional claims, not merely to a starburst or highlighted flag. Stacking claims related to a specific healthy issue, i.e. coronary health, was highly effective for eliciting consumer reac-

W. Loh

TABLE 7.1
Summary of Consumer Response to Breakfast Cereal Survey

			Everyone		Buyers only	
Total Surveyed		100				
Respondents		67	67%			
Buy cereals?	YES	64	96%			
	NO	3	4%			
Preference	Box A	9	15%		8	14%
	Box B	51	85%		49	86%
Price for Box B?	<$3.09	1	2%		1	2%
	$3.09	38	60%		36	60%
	>$3.09–$3.39	14	22%		13	22%
	>$3.39–$3.69	7	11%		7	12%
	>$3.69 - $3.99	1	2%		1	2%
	>$3.99	2	3%		2	3%
		Box A	Box B		Box A	Box B
Reason? (Unaided)	Appearance	4	1		4	1
	Health	2	51		2	49
	Taste	3	0		2	0

tion. Listing only a single claim or a multiplicity of unrelated claims, e.g. folic acid supplementation and high calcium, was less effective. One can speculate that the consumer perceives higher benefits for specific disease issues when multiple claims exist, although more detailed analyses would be required for proof.

At this writing, the FDA has not yet provided guidelines on a health claim relating to *trans* fat. The "zero *trans* fat" claim used in this test is not yet legal. However, the FDA has exercised its discretionary enforcement authority to permit the statement "0 gm of *trans* fat" on the front of many food products. It has not enforced regulations against those companies that list "No Trans Fat" on their products.

How to Reformulate?

The manner by which consumers react to front of the package nutrition claims present an opportunity to deliver higher value to the consumer and, by doing so, provide an opportunity to extract greater value in the form of increased market share and/or higher price point. Methodical testing of consumer reaction can determine which claims do or do not work. How will the consumer react if only one, or at most two, claims can be justified? If no front of the package claims are possible, will improvements to the Nutrition Fact panel or the ingredient statement deliver any perceived consumer value? Just by testing various packaging designs, those benefits that the consumer values the most can be identified and prioritized. It is those specific benefits that must justify the decision for reformulation.

Since multiple brands compete in the marketplace, competitive scenarios must be tested. How would your customers react if a competitor brand was relaunched with front of the package nutritional claims? What would be its impact on relative market share and price? Will the "healthier" brand command a higher price point or will the "less healthy" brand be forced to a lower price point? Equally important is the impact of reformulation on brand equity. Does the consumer expect your brand to offer the "healthy" option? If not, there may be no reason to proceed with reformulation.

In addition to a comprehensive analysis of marketplace reaction to different product concepts, related business issues have to be considered. Is the brand likely to draw the attention of activist groups? Will the brand be singled out for adverse media attention, including the unrelenting eye of cable news? How will stock analysts react to a *trans* fat reformulation, or lack of one, in branded products owned by public companies?

The cost of reformulation, although it can vary widely among product categories, will be significant. The financial impact of *trans* reformulation, both positive and negative, has to be calculated first. The positive impact on market share, price, and potential leverage for retail shelf space has to be weighed against the impact of development cost, higher manufacturing cost and potential dilution of brand equity. *Trans* reformulation should proceed if the net calculation is positive and the cost of the reformulation effort reflects an acceptable return on investment.

Most food companies calculating the cost of reformulation focus primarily on increased oil cost. Since hydrogenated soybean oil was widely adopted by the industry for more than thirty years, competitive pressures have inexorably improved system efficiency. Any option other than partially hydrogenated soybean oil will be delivered by a less efficient system and cost more, at least at the outset. New oils that deliver reduced and zero *trans* fat statements are in short supply. Demand will inevitably drive higher price until supply and demand balance.

The first product line targeted for reformulation is typically the most important brand. For many companies, a heritage brand is the single most valuable asset of the company. This is an asset that consistently delivers a set of consumer benefits and in turn provides the brand owner with a reliable source of cash. Often, the exact consumer benefit is hard to quantify. Over time, however, such brands acquire an aura of personal security.

Food companies may work to lower supply chain costs and increase manufacturing productivity, but no changes can be made to the visual or organoleptic characteristics of the branded product or product line. If the data from consumer focus studies however point to reformulation, making changes to the heritage brand becomes the top priority.

To date, the food companies undergoing reformulation have directed very significant R&D resources to the effort. In the majority of cases, however, there are no "drop-in" substitutes. The chance that a "zero *trans*" oil will replace the original shortening without impacting product taste, appearance, shelf life or other related functionality is remote. Reducing or eliminating *trans* fat in processed foods may involve having to change the recipe, the manufacturing process and even the packaging system.

Because the stakes are so high for a strong brand, the reformulation process will be closely monitored and scrutinized. Following reformulation, the level of testing is usually higher than new product launches. In the ideal situation, the consumer should not be able to discern any difference in the product before and after reformulation. To do so requires very intensive testing and most companies have not programmed sufficient time for consumer testing following reformulation.

If the functionality of the replacement oil does not exactly match that of the original oil, then the product may have different features. A cookie may have greater spread or less rise, depending on the choice of replacement shortening. Fat content may have to be reduced or replaced by other food ingredients. The manufacturing process may have to be changed, requiring capital expenditures. The shelf life stability of the product may be altered, requiring changes to the packaging material. The new recipe has to withstand environmental fluctuations, including temperature, humidity and mechanical pressure, during warehousing and delivery.

Should the packaging incorporate health claims on front of the package? If the *trans* reformulation process was properly planned, that question should have been answered in the initial consumer focus studies. If not, then consumer research will be required to define and test the appropriate positioning for the reformulated product. New packaging film will have to be ordered and the transition from old film to new film will have to be coordinated with the transition from the old recipe to the new one.

Food companies with multiple brands face even more challenging issues. A single plant may produce multiple branded stock-keeping units (SKU). The pressure to reduce costs every year usually results in gradual conversion of all the recipes to standard ingredients, including oil. Many food manufacturing plants produce multiple products using a single oil—and have only one oil tank. If only some brands are scheduled for reformulation, then additional tanks and piping will have to be installed to accommodate one or more new oils. Food companies with multiple brands will also have to manage the transition of some brands to a reduced or zero *trans* status before their other brands convert.

How Not to Reformulate?

With less than nine months to go before the *trans* fat labeling deadline, many food companies are still working on product reformulation. Some will succeed and others will not. Those reformulation efforts driven by the product development function are usually among the less successful. Without close collaboration with the marketing function to define those reformulation objectives that maximize consumer benefits, *trans* reformulation usually takes longer and requires larger investments.

Such reformulation efforts begin by asking oil suppliers for advice on various options for *trans* reformulation. This process, however, ignores the most important opinion—that of the customer. Oil suppliers cannot provide advice on what a food company's customers want. That information can only come from the customers.

Depending on the product segment and the brand image, consumers can have very different expectations for nutrition.

Unless the consumer can be engaged to provide their perspective on the brand, the value of a reformulation effort cannot be determined. Reformulation of core brands represents a huge corporate investment, one that should be justified on the basis of return on investment. The cost of reformulation should be compared against measurable returns from the reformulated product, either to maintain or increase market share, maintaining or increase selling price. The cost of capital investments has to be added to the formula. Alternatively, the impact of non-reformulation has to be assessed. Will competitive products reformulate and impact market share and/or selling price? Will the brand be targeted for adverse publicity? How will Wall Street react to the reformulation decision?

In order to proceed, the cost of reformulation and the anticipated benefits must outweigh the impact of not reformulating. Otherwise, there may be no reason to reduce or eliminate *trans* fat. FDA labeling regulations do not require that food products become "*trans* free," only that their *trans* fat content be disclosed. If disclosure of *trans* fat does not materially impact consumer perception of a particular brand, then the need to reformulate is greatly lessened.

Epilogue

Several events have joined to create "perfect storm" that has made nutrition a potential driver for the food industry. While consumers have always made purchasing decisions on the basis of taste and convenience, the value of superior nutrition appears to be tangible and quantifiable. Health, like taste and convenience, may have become a major driver for consumer choice. However, the consumer's perception of nutritional improvements can differ by product category. A decision to reduce or eliminate *trans* fatty acid content in branded products should rely on quantifiable measures of perceived benefit.

Reduced *trans* or *trans* free status is only one of many factors that contribute to a healthier perception of a branded product. A common strategy using off shore oils involves eliminating *trans* fatty acids at the expense of increasing saturated fat. How will consumers react to shifting the values in the Nutrition Fact panel? What is the tradeoff from eliminating *trans* fat while listing tropical oils in the ingredient statement? The only way to know is to ask the consumer. Their response may differ by product, brand promise and product category.

While this article focused purely on *trans* labeling in the United States, the rest of the world is changing as well. As of March of 2005, Israel becomes the fifth nation to require disclosure of *trans* fat in processed foods, with the ultimate objective of eliminating them. Australia, Canada, Denmark and the United States have already taken different measures to disclose and/or eliminate *trans* fat from the diet. The European Commission has asked the European Food Safety Authority for a scientific opinion on the role of *trans* fats in human health. The trend is toward more regulation of *trans* fat, not less.

Appendix

Commercial Solutions

Introduction

Since the July 2003 announcement of the Food and Drug Administration (FDA), requiring food nutrition labels to contain *trans* fats, food manufacturers have devoted a considerable amount of resources to find alternate solutions. The new regulations do not require reformulating the food products to reduce or eliminate the *trans* fats, but do require a disclosure of *trans* fat content along with saturated fat on the "Nutrition Facts" label. Even though many food products we consume have contained *trans* fats for decades, the current media attention is influencing a negative consumer perception of *trans* fat. In effect, most of the food manufacturers would like to have their products contain no or little *trans* fats. The food product manufacturers want to make the necessary modifications to their products by the FDA's required deadline of January 1, 2006. Due to a number of steps involved, such as new ingredient supply logistics, processing, labeling etc. they need to make the decision to choose from various reformulation options at least 6 months ahead of this date.

As stated in chapter 7, defining the business objective should precede the technical reformulation of a product. There are a number of technical options available for food manufacturers to reformulate their products with alternate fat or oil ingredients. However, most of the alternate ingredients have their own drawbacks such as higher cost, lower functionality and shelf life. For example, choosing a palm fraction to replace the hydrogenated fat may increase the saturated fat and also requires including palm oil as one of the ingredients. As a result, the food manufacturers must sort through all these options and balance the risk/reward ratio before making their decision. Choosing alternate ingredients also requires an understanding of the composition, characteristics and the resulting features and benefits. Finally, the chosen ingredients need to be evaluated in the food product by a sensory panel for consumer satisfaction.

To provide the information on the state-of-the-art *trans* fats solutions to our readers, we requested the commercial solutions from the fats and oils suppliers that they are currently offering to their customers. We compiled the following information provided by the fats and oils suppliers as *trans* fats reduction/elimination solutions with limited editing.

Aarhus United USA

Aarhus United has developed three families of non-hydrogenated, zero-*trans* products. These products are all based on naturally occurring solids found in vegetable oils. These products are not just alternatives to products made from partially hydrogenated vegetable oils, they should be considered alternatives for the generation of products, which preceded hydrogenation: butter fat, lard, and cocoa butter.

Butterfat and lard owe their unique characteristics to the high number of different triglycerides, which melt over a broad range of temperatures. The broad range of fatty acids needed to reproduce the characteristics of the animal fats however are not all from the same source. Naturally solid fats such as palm (and its many fractions), palm kernel and coconut oils along with various soft oils are the source of these various fatty acids and triglycerides needed. The characteristics needed for specific applications are obtained through blending and the co-interesterification of various blends of whole oils and specific fractions of oils. Aarhus United's EsSense and Cisao families of products were developed as highly functional margarines, shortenings, and margarine hard stocks.

EsSense

EsSense products are margarine and shortening oils designed to meet the demands of *trans* elimination while maintaining a low level of saturated fat also (Table 1). The challenges of these objectives go beyond the formulation of triglycerides: it involves the need for possible processing changes and careful handling by the customer. The rugged characteristics of a fat system high in the combination of solids form both saturated fat and *trans* fat are replaced with a solid matrix comprised of specific fat crystals capable of entraining more liquid components. The applications for EsSense have moved beyond margarine. With the utilization of high stability oils as the liquid portion of the blend, members of this family are now used as spray oils by the baking industry.

TABLE 1
Zero *trans*, Non-Hydrogenated & "Low Saturates"

	EsSence™			
	86-23	86-33	86-43	86-53
Mettler Drop Point °F	94-99	99-104	106-112	108-114
% *trans*	<1	<1	<1	<1
% Saturated	20	24	33	40
% Monounsaturated	55	52	46	42
% Polyunsaturated	24	23	20	17

The EsSense line is based on a hard stock base blended with liquid oil. In addition low saturates and zero *trans* fat, these products can be formulated with the liquid oil of the choice, allowing a company to "customize" it for a source oil of their choice.

Cisao

A family of rugged shortenings with zero *trans* and/or no hydrogenated components, the Cisao products cover a wide range of melting points. In addition to bakery shortenings, pastry applications, and frying fats these products are also used as filling fats in cream cookies and icings. Cisao products also display good crystallization and melting properties and are non-tempering (Table 2).

Cebes®NH

Cocoa butter alternatives from lauric oils have always been very low in *trans* fat. The desire to eliminate the word "hydrogenation" from labels entirely has presented challenges. In the past and with today's high speed processing demands, a fully hydrogenated palm oil had been used to help start crystallization of cocoa butter substitutes. Today, through the selection of very special fractions of palm kernel and palm, a non-hydrogenated and non-tempering group of confectionery fats have been developed. The Cebes® NH family has been expanded to incorporate the special needs from this group of fats.

TABLE 2
Zero *trans* & Non-Hydrogenated

	Cisao®			
	78-20	81-36	83-12	83-67
Mettler Drop Point °F	95-100	115-121	103-110	80-84
IV	20-30	46-52	50-60	55
SFC @	%	%	%	%
10°C	69-73	57-63	51-55	35-39
20°C	40-44	35-41	29-33	3-7
30°C	11-16	15-20	9-13	0
40°C	<5	6-12	1-3	0
% *trans*	<1	<1	<1	<1
% Sats	78	54	48	48
% Mono	19	37	40	40
Labeling Code	A	B	B	B

A, Palm and Palm Kernel Oil
B, Palm Oil

TABLE 3
Cebes®NH (Non-Hydrogenated) & Zero *trans*

	Cebes®			
	29-01NH	29-02NH	29-04NH	29-07NH
Mettler Drop Point °F	94-98	96-100	101-104	104-108
% *trans*	<1	<1	<1	<1
% Saturated	91.8	98.3	95.1	92.0
% Monounsaturated	7.0	5.0	4.0	7.0
% Polyunsaturated	1.0	1.0	0.7	0.8

Now you can formulate coatings that are non-hydrogenated and zero *trans*. For the first time, Aarhus can offer you a product with these attributes over a variety of melt points to fit your current market demand (Table 3).

Ed Wilson
Aarhus United USA
131 Marsh St.
Port Newark, NJ 07114
ed.wilson@aarhusunited.com

ADM NovaLipids

ADM is pleased to contribute to the development of low *trans* solutions for food applications. ADM Food Oils is providing functional low *trans* alternatives by taking a four-pronged approach. These four areas of lipid technology include Naturally Stable Oils; Lauric and Palm Fats; Blended Fats and Oils; and Enzyme Interesterified Shortenings and Margarine.

These areas of interest address the functionality and stability issues of low *trans* product development. ADM is continually striving to develop new technologies that can utilize domestic sources of fats and oils, which can provide the most functional and economic products possible.

Naturally Stable Oils

Naturally stable oils are typically oils that contain low levels of linolenic acid. Cottonseed oil, corn oil and mid pleic sunflower oil are all low in linolenic acid, therefore these oils do not require partial hydrogenation to reduce the negative oxidative effects of linolenic acid. These oils can be used alone or in blends for food applications such as frying, spray oils or even in limited baking applications. Naturally stable oils are also being evaluated in the development of enzymatically interesterified shortenings and margarines. The list of these oils is seen in the Table 1.

Lauric and Palm Fats

Lauric fats are very useful for coating and spray oil applications. These products are very high in saturated fatty acids, but are very functional and exhibit excellent inherent stability. ADM currently supplies coconut, hydrogenated coconut, palm kernel and hydrogenated palm kernel oils. ADM also introduced the first enzymatically interesterified palm kernel oil confectionary fat to the North American market in 2002. This product (95°F PK) is also a good substitute for high *trans* cocoa butter replacers. For low *trans* developmental work these products can be used alone or as part of a blend. Tables 2 and 3 contain typical analysis of neat and modified lauric fats.

Palm oil and palm fractions are also are being utilized in the development of low *trans* shortenings and margarine. Both palm oil and palm fractions can be blended with domestic oils such as soybean oil to reduce saturates and improve functional

TABLE 1
Fatty Acid Composition of Naturally Stable Oils

Oil	C16:0	C18:0	C18:1	C18:2	C18:3	*trans*
Corn Oil	11.3	2.0	28.0	56.5	<1.0	<1.5%
Cottonseed Oil	23.5	2.4	16.3	55.0	<1.0	<1.5%
Nusun	4.6	3.7	60.5	28.6	<1.0	<1.5%

TABLE 2
Typical Analysis of Palm Kernel Based Fats

Analysis	Palm Kernel Oil	PH Palm Kernel	H Palm Kernel	PH Re Palm K	PH Re Palm K
MDP F	78-84	103-109	110-114	95-98	101-103
IV	15-21	3-6	4 max.	4 max.	4 max.
SFI 50 F	65-74	67-73	68-75	64-69	68-75
SFI 70 F	28-39	57-63	64-70	53-57	54-60
SFI 80 F	15 max.	37-43	46-52	36-42	40-45
SFI 92 F	1 max.	—	18-24	8-12	11-15
SFI 104 F	0	2-6	8-14	0	4 max.
Total TFA (%)	1.5	4	1.5	3	3
Total Saturates (%)	83.8	96.5	99.5	96.3	96.5

TABLE 3
Typical Analysis of Coconut Oil Based Fats

Analysis	Coconut	H Coconut	H Coconut + H Soy	H Coconut + H Soy
MDP F	72.0-78.0	93.0-97.0	98.0-102.0	103.0-108.0
IV	7-11	1.5 max.	1.5 max.	5 max.
SFI 50 F	52-58	61-67	61-67	61-70
SFI 70 F	23-29	37-43	38-44	38-44
SFI 80 F	1 max.	9-15	9-15	—
SFI 92 F	0	4 max.	3-9	3-9
SFI 104 F	—	1 max.	4 max.	2-8
Total TFA	< 2	< 2	< 2	< 2
Total Saturates	92	98	98	98

attributes. These blends can be used in a variety of baking applications where low *trans* solid fat requirements are needed. Table 4 contains the data for various blend ratios of palm oil and soybean oil.

Blending

Blending of fats and oils is an area where a wide array of options can be utilized. Solutions can include the blending of oils such as soy, corn, cotton and Nusun with fully hydrogenated soybean and or cottonseed oil to produce a fluid type shortening. Fluid shortenings can be used in a variety of applications in the bakery. Various degrees of solidification can be achieved depending on the level of hard stock added. Another aspect of blending is to produce blends of brush hydrogenated soybean oil with naturally stable oils. These oil blends can be used for a variety of applications which include frying and spray oils. Even though partially hydrogenated soybean oil is a component of the blend, and taking into account the amount of fat per serving, the level of *trans* can be minimized to claim less than 0.5g of *trans* per serving and therefore "0" grams *trans* per serving. Table 5 lists blends designed for par-frying or QSR frying.

Appendix

TABLE 4
Palm Oil / Soybean Oil Blends

Analysis	Palm	90% Palm 10% SBO	80% Palm 20% SBO	70% SBO 30% SBO	60% Palm 40% SBO	50% Palm 50% SBO
SFI 50F	37.6	29.5	24.9	19.1	14.2	10.2
SFI 70F	17.2	12.4	10.6	7.8	6.1	5.1
SFI 80F	14.1	10.4	9.0	6.6	5.2	4.4
SFI 92F	8.4	8.3	6.9	5.0	3.6	3.3
SFI 104F	4.2	4.9	4.2	2.6	1.3	1.2
MDP F	105.3	102.0	99.1	98.9	96.8	93.7
%C16:0	44.0	40.6	37.3	33.8	30.4	27.2
%C18:0	4.3	4.3	4.3	4.3	4.3	4.3
%C18:1	40.0	31.2	35.9	34.5	32.9	31.3
%C18:2	9.1	13.5	13.5	22.1	26.4	30.5
%C18:3	0.3	1.0	1.8	2.6	3.3	4.0
% Total Sats.	51.2	47.6	44.1	40.4	36.9	33.5
%Total *trans*	0.6	0.6	0.6	0.6	0.6	0.6

TABLE 5
Typical Analysis of Low *trans* Blended Lipid Systems

Fatty Acid	70% Nusun / 30% PHSBO	70% Cottonseed 30% PHSBO	70% Corn / 30% PHSBO
Total C16:0	6.1	19.2	10.9
Total C18:0	4.6	3.8	3.5
Total C18:1	52.9	21.6	29.6
Total C18:2	32.2	50.7	52.0
Total C18:3 cis	1.7	1.6	2.1
Total *trans*	<3.4	<3.4	<3.4
Total Saturates	12.4	24.6	15.5

Enzymatic Interesterification

Enzyme interesterified shortening and margarine product development and production is an area that ADM has pioneered. ADM currently commercializes a variety of products using immobilized lipase technology, such as 95°F palm kernel oil as well as enzymatically interesterified domestic blends of soybean oil and hydrogenated soybean oil used as margarine, spread and shortening base-stocks. The domestic products mentioned above are typically produced from enzymatically interesterifying a blend of soybean oil and fully hydrogenated soybean oil. By varying the level of fully hydrogenated vegetable oil (hardstock) in the blend we can modify the melting and functional characteristics of the shortening or margarine. The fully hydrogenated soybean oil used in these blends is completely saturated, therefore minimizing *trans* isomer formation. Table 6 lists the various solid fat profiles that can be achieved by interesterifying soybean oil with fully hydrogenated soybean oil.

TABLE 6
Enzymatically Interesterified Blends of Soybean Oil

Analysis	10%	15%	20%	25%	30%	35% Titer[a]	40%	45%	50%	55%	60%
SFI @ 50	2.8	7.1	11.9	16.9	22	27.3	33	40.1	46.8	52.1	55.9
SFI @ 70	1.4	3.2	5	7.6	11.1	15.7	20.6	26.9	34.9	40.8	44.5
SFI @ 80	1	2.9	4.4	6.7	10	14.4	19.2	25.4	34.1	39.5	41.2
SFI @ 92	0.2	2	3.1	5.7	8.5	12.6	17	22.9	30.9	34.9	35.8
SFI @ 104	0	1.4	1.3	2.9	5.9	9.5	13.1	18.3	25.1	29.2	30

[a]Titer = fully hydrogenated soybean oil.

Enzymatic interesterified shortenings and margarines utilizing soybean oil and fully hydrogenated soybean oil tend to be rich in stearic, omega-6 and omega-3 fatty acids. The American Heart Association has indicated that stearic acid may not affect or may even lower blood cholesterol. When soybean oil is used as the liquid portion of the blend the levels of omega-3 and omega-6 fatty acids are also increased compared to palm oil or partially hydrogenated vegetable oils used for similar applications. ADM has also received notification from the FDA that when foods are formulated with interesterified soybean oil, the descriptor of "interesterified soybean oil" can be used in the ingredient statement.

For questions or comments regarding ADM NovaLipid products, feel free to visit admworld.com.

Mark Matlock
Archer Daniels Midland Co.
1001 N. Brush College Road
Decatur, IL 62521-1656
Matlock@ADMWORLD.com

Bunge Oils

As one of the leading edible oil suppliers in North America, with facilities located across the United States and Canada, Bunge is well positioned to offer a broad range of *trans* Reduction Options. Bunge offers options utilizing proprietary hydrogenation, palm and lauric oils, and new oilseed varieties possessing unique traits.

Presently Food Processors are faced with the challenge of providing high quality, good tasting products and trying to predict what the actual consumer perception of *trans* fatty acids will be. With consumer perception being what it is, it is extremely difficult to forecast what the most desirable option for *trans* reduction is for 2006 and beyond. For that reason, Bunge has invested significant research efforts into developing technologies and products that address three primary customer needs:

- Reduction of *trans* fatty acids with minimal increase in saturates
- Reduction in *trans* and elimination of hydrogenation from the label
- Reduction in *trans* / elimination of hydrogenation and no tropical oils

Bunge's portfolio of offerings for *trans* fatty acid reduction is expanding rapidly. An overview of some of the products available is provided here.

RighT Line of Products

For customers who have chosen to reduce the *trans* fatty acids in their products but do not wish to significantly increase the saturated fatty acid levels, Bunge has developed the *RighT* line of products. Bunge's *RighT* line of products are based upon a proprietary hydrogenation process using domestic oil sources.

Vream *RighT* ™ All Purpose Shortening
- 80% Reduction in *trans* vs Standard All Purpose
- 33% Reduction in the sum of *trans* + Saturates
- Drop-in replacement in many All Purpose Applications including Cookies, Biscuits, Pie Crusts, Tortillas and Mixes.

Vreamay *RighT* ™ Cake and Icing Shortening
- 80% Reduction in *trans* vs Standard Cake and Icing Shortening
- 33% Reduction in the sum of *trans* + Saturates
- Drop-in replacement in many Cake & Icing Applications

Victor *RighT* ™ Margarine
- 80% Reduction in *trans* vs Standard Bakers Grade Margarine
- 33% Reduction in the sum of *trans* + Saturates
- Drop-in replacement in many All Purpose Margarine Applications including Danish, Cookies, Icings and Fillings.

Other specialized margarines and emulsified shortenings based upon the *RighT* Technology are constantly being added to the product line.

NH Line of Products

For customers who want to reduce the *trans* fatty acids in their products and have a need to remove "hydrogenated" from their ingredient statement, Bunge offers the NH Line of products. These products are specially formulated primarily from palm and palm kernel oils. Many of the Bunge Shortenings available for years are now available in the NH line of products.

- Vream® NH All Purpose Shortening
- Vreamay® NH Cake & Icing Shortening
- Cremol® NH Specialty Icing Shortening
- Super Cel® NH Specialty Cake Shortening
- Victor® NH Bakers Grade Margarine
- Croissant NH Margarine
- Coral ® NH Margarine
- Summit® 40 NH Butter Blend Margarine
- Bakers Ideal® NH Pastry Margarine
- Anhydrous NH Roll-In Shortening
- NH Biscuit Flakes
- Tri-Co® NH Emulsified Dough Shortening

Other NH products can be tailored to the specific functional and nutritional needs of the food processor. While removing *trans* fatty acids and eliminating hydrogenation is important, some processors are also concerned about the level of saturated fatty acids in their products. For that reason, Bunge is offering functional products covering a wide range of saturated fatty acid contents.

Specialty Oils

For applications where a lightly hydrogenated oil has been used in the past, Bunge is offering oils that have been developed for higher stability without need of hydrogenation. These oils are suitable as spray oils, frying oils and for blending in many other applications.

Nutra Clear HS™ Canola Oil

Bunge, the leading producer of canola oil in North America continues to bring new canola products to market with the introduction of Nutra Clear HS ™ Canola Oil, a specially bred, nonhydrogenated high stability oil developed for use in various applications such as salad dressings, cracker and snack spray oil, cooking and frying.

NUTRIUM™ Low Linolenic Soybean Oil

Bunge and Dupont are leading the way into the next generation of soybean oil with the launch of NUTRIUM Low Linolenic Soybean Oil, a low linolenic soybean oil designed for applications such as salad dressings, cracker and snack spray oil, cooking and frying..

Contact Bunge

The needs of the market are changing rapidly and so are Bunge's trans reduction offerings. For the most up-to-date offerings contact Bunge at www.bungeoils.com.

NUTRIUM™ is a trademark of Pioneer Hi-Bred International, Inc.

Bob Johnson
Bunge Oils
725 N. Kinzie Ave.
Bradley, IL 60914
Bob.Johnson@Bunge.com

Cargill Specialty Oils

Cargill Specialty Oils offer a complete line of zero *trans*, high stability oils. These new generation oils deliver exceptional stability without hydrogenation. These oils deliver superior food flavor, unmatched convenience and outstanding performance.

Zero *trans* Liquid Oils

High oleic canola oils have been specially developed by Cargill scientists to deliver high heat and oxidative stability without hydrogenation. By changing the fatty acid compositions of these oils, there is an increased resistance to oxidation, thus, the development of off-odors and flavors are prevented. Cargill Specialty Oils also offer a line of high oleic sunflower oil, which has zero *trans* from hydrogenation. The fatty acid composition and the oxidative stability of these oils in comparison to standard canola are shown in Table 1.

Cargill also offers higher stability liquid oils with natural antioxidants. The fatty acid composition and the oxidative stability of these oils are provided in Table 2 below.

TABLE 1

Typical Fatty Acid Composition and Specifications of High Oleic Canola and Sunflower Oils

	Standard Canola	Clear Valley 65	Clear Valley 75	Clear Valley High Oleic Sunflower
C16:0, Palmitic	4%	4%	4%	4%
C18:0, Stearic	2%	2%	2%	4%
C18:1, Oleic	58%	65%	74%	79%
C18:2, Linoleic	26%	22%	12%	11%
C18:3, Linolenic	10%	3%	4%	<0.5%
Total *trans*	1.5	1.5% max	1.5% max	1.5% max
Total Sats.	7	7%	7%	8%
AOM Hours	12	25 min	34 min	35 min

TABLE 2

Fatty Acid Composition and Oxidative Stability of High Stability Oils

	Odyssey 95	Odyssey 100
C16:0, Palmitic	4%	4%
C18:0, Stearic	2%	4%
C18:1, Oleica	65%	79%
C18:2, Linoleic	22%	11%
C18:3, Linolenic	3%	<0.5%
Total *trans*	1.5% max	1.5% max
Total Sats.	7%	7%
AOM Hours	95 min	100 min

Zero *trans* Solid Shortenings

The following shortenings were developed to meet demanding applications that require solids without increasing saturated fats. Cargill's TransEND· line exhibits superior functionality to meet the requirements of solids shortenings with essentially zero *trans* fat. TransEND 350 is a soft *zero trans* solid shortening developed for the manufacture of cookies, crackers, breads, pizza dough, scones and cake mixes. TransEND 370 is a *zero trans* solid shortening developed for the manufacture of cookies, biscuits, dough mix and doughnuts. TransEND 390 is a relatively hard *zero trans* solid shortening developed for the manufacture of pastries, biscuits and piecrusts. The specifications of TransEnd line of products are shown in Table 3.

The solid fat profiles of TransEnd products do not match the conventional shortentings. The functionality and mouth feel of TransEnd products are tested in various food applications. The solid fat index, % at various temperatures are shown in Table 4.

For further information regarding the above products, feel free to visit www.clearvalleyoils.com.

TABLE 3
The Specifications of TransEnd Line of Products

	TransEND® 350	TransEND® 370	TransEND® 390
Total Sats	10%-14%	13%-17%	18%-22%
Total Trans	2% max	2% max	2% max
AOM Hours	70 min	80 min	85 min
Mettler Drop Point	109-114°F	112-120°F	123-130°F

TABLE 4
The Solid Fat Index, % at Different Temperatures of TransEnd Products

Solid Fat Index	TransEND, 350	TransEND, 370	TransEND, 390
@ 50°F, %	5.5–9.0	7.5–12.0	13.0–18.0
@ 70°F, %	4.5–7.5	6.0–10.0	11.0–16.0
@ 90°F, %	3.0–6.0	4.0–8.0	9.0–13.0
@ 104°F, %	2.0–4.5	3.0–6.0	7.0–9.5

Willie H. Loh
Cargill Specialty Canola Oils
P.O. Box 5693/Lake
Minneapolis, MN 55417
willie_loh@cargill.com

Loders Croklaan

Palm Oil: A Versatile and Cost Effective Alternative to *trans* Fat

Palm oil is obtained from the fruit of the oil palm, a tree that grows within 10 degrees of the equator. Annual global production of palm oil is approximately 50 billion pounds, second only to soybean oil. The majority of world production comes from Malaysia and Indonesia, most of which is traded as a commodity. Loders Croklaan's parent company, IOI, is the largest privately held producer and refiner of palm oil in Malaysia. The top three users of palm oil are the European Union, India and China, with about 85% of the oil being used in food manufacture. Palm fruit is composed of a fleshy outer layer that contains the palm oil, and a hard kernel that has smaller amount of a different oil called palm kernel oil. Palm oil consists mainly of palmitic and oleic acids, which are the two main fatty acids found in the human body. Palm kernel oil contains a high level of lauric acid which imparts unique physical properties to this fat.

Supply and Cost

Palm oil supplies about 25% of the world's edible oil, second only to soybean oil at about 30%, while palm oil is the most traded edible oil. Large supply chains are already in place throughout the world and Loders Croklaan is a major palm oil importer in Europe. Loders Croklaan's parent company is the largest privately held palm oil producer in Malaysia. Palm oil prices are closely linked to soybean oil prices and palm is cost neutral to soy averaged over time.

Palm Oil Functionality

Palm oil is recognized throughout the world as an excellent fat for almost any food application, without the need for hydrogenation. The European Union uses approximately six billion pounds per year in a wide variety of foodstuffs, similar to the processed and fried foods used in the U.S. today. The key to a successful baking fat is its ability to naturally crystallize in a stable form called beta-prime. This crystal form is small in size and imparts a smooth texture to the fat, allowing easy blending with dry ingredients. These crystals efficiently entrap small air bubbles, a critical requirement in many products that require creaming for their functionality. Palmitic acid, the main saturated fat in palm oil, naturally crystallizes in the beta-prime form, making palm oil an excellent substitute for *trans* fat. Another benefit of palmitic acid is that its beta-prime form is stable. This means that the finished product will retain its aerated volume and creamy texture over extended periods of storage. Palm oil is also naturally stable without hydrogenation as it contains no linolenic acid and a low level of linoleic acid. This provides extended shelf life to food products, the same as found with hydrogenated fats. Palm oil can be converted into many different products through the process of fractionation. Multiple fractions can be blended together or with other oils to offer almost any match to *trans*-containing fats. Loders Croklaan has over 100 years of experience in the processing and fractionation of palm oil.

Palm Oil Products

Loders Croklaan currently offers over 30 products based on palm oil, in bulk, cubed and flaked forms. All products are free of *trans* fat and are non-hydrogenated. This guarantees that all finished products will read 0g *trans* fat on the nutrition panel in conformity to FDA labeling requirements. The terms "hydrogenated" or "partially hydrogenated" will not appear on the ingredient statement, an advantage to the food manufacturer as these terms are often perceived by consumers as synonymous with *trans* fat. Loders Croklaan creates a wide diversity of products by combining a broad range of different palm fractions and in some cases by applying its long established interesterification process. The products are further tailor made by blending with liquid oils such as sunflower or soybean oils.

The products range is divided into 2 main brands. *Sanstrans* oils and shortenings, and *Freedom* coating fats. Loders also offers Durkex NT 100, a high stability liquid oil for specialty applications.

The *Sanstrans* range contains several standard shortenings of varying hardness and melting points that can be used in large numbers of applications (Table 1). The products are distinguished by a number that indicates the approximate melting point in degrees Celsius, therefore products with higher numbers are generally harder. In general these products are the lowest cost palm option, having the same functionality as the most commonly used partially hydrogenated vegetable oil shortenings in use today. *Sanstrans* 39, *Sanstrans* 42 and *Sanstrans* 45 are a close match to the hydrogenated all-purpose cake and cookie shortenings commonly used in the food industry

TABLE 1
Sanstrans Standard Bakery Shortenings and Fats

Product	Melting point (°C/°F)	Type	Typical applications
Sanstrans 55	55/131	Hard structuring fat	Dry mix, icing stabilizer, heat stability improver
Sanstrans 50	50/122	Hard structuring fat	Structuring fat
Sanstrans 45	45/113	Hard plastic shortening	Cookies and crackers
Sanstrans 42	42/108	Plastic shortening	All purpose shortening
Sanstrans 39	39/102	Soft plastic shortening	Cakes, cookies and fillers
Sanstrans 35	35/95	Soft plastic shortening	Dairy substitute
Sanstrans 25	25/77	Fluid oil	Industrial and food service applications requiring a fluid oil

today. We commissioned the American Institute of Baking (AIB) to evaluate *Sanstrans* 39 and *Sanstrans* 45 side by side with hydrogenated shortening in a cookie and yellow cake applications. The AIB used its own standard formulas and conditions for sugar snap cookies and yellow cake without adjustment. The results, shown in figure 1, demonstrate that performance was essentially identical between the 2 fats types (*Sanstrans* 39 for yellow cake and *Sanstrans* 45 for cookies).

Table 2 shows frying oils and shortenings currently available from Loders Croklaan. Palm oil is naturally stable in frying without the need for hydrogenation, as it contains no linolenic acid and has a low level of linoleic acid. *Sanstrans* Liquid Fry is a suitable alternative to a low solids, fluid hydrogenated frying oil. *Sanstrans* Fry is similar in stability and performance to high *trans*, hydrogenated shortenings. Several hydrogenated donut frying shortenings with differing performance characteristics are used in the U.S. at present and Loders Croklaan manufactures a number of no-*trans* palm-based options that match these products. The standard low cost product for general use is *Sanstrans* Donut Fry P, while *Sanstrans* DD results in a less oily donut, ideal where high quality sugar coating is desired. For situations where a neutral odor during frying is required, Loders Croklaan offers *Sanstrans* DDC.

Loders Croklaan has combined its current line of food grade emulsifiers with palm oil to offer a range of no-*trans*, non-hydrogenated emulsified shortenings. The products shown in Table 3 cover the most common applications for emulsified shortenings, and will give similar performance with minimal adjustment to process conditions.

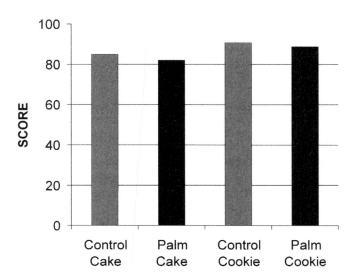

Fig. 1. Comparison of palm-based shortenings and *trans*-containing control shortening in yellow cake and sugar snap cookies, using identical formulas and conditions. Palm Cake = Sanstrans 39; Palm cookie = Sanstrans 45. Quality scores were essentially the same for control and palm oil.

TABLE 2
Sanstrans Frying Fats and Oils[a]

Product	Melting point (°C/°F)	Type	Typical applications
Sanstrans Fry	48/118	Plastic shortening	General purpose frying fat in cubes
Sanstrans Bulk Fry	48/118	Liquid	General purpose frying fat in bulk tankers
Sanstrans Liquid Fry	25/77	Fluid oil	Fluid, general purpose frying oil
Sanstrans Donut Fry P	48/118	Plastic shortening	Standard donut frying fat
Sanstrans DD	47/116	Plastic shortening	Reduced oiliness donut frying fat
Sanstrans DDC	45/113	Plastic shortening	Flavor modified donut frying fat

[a]All frying oils and fats contain silicone except for donut frying fats.

TABLE 3
Sanstrans Emulsified Shortenings

Product	Emulsifiers	Typical applications
Sanstrans Icing Shortening	Mono/di-glycerides and Polysorbate 60	Cake icings
Sanstrans Soft Icing Shortening	Mono/di-glycerides and Polysorbate 60	Creamy icings, scoopable
Sanstrans Cake Shortening	Mono/di-glycerides,	Excellent aeration in cakes
Sanstrans Cakemix	Mono/di-glycerides, PGME and lecithin	Formulated for use in packaged cake mixes
Sanstrans Perflex	Mono/di-glycerides, PGME and lecithin	High potency for lower use rate of shortening in all cake types

Table 4 shows the *Freedom* line of no-*trans*, non-hydrogenated coating fats. Loders Croklaan has an existing portfolio of coating fats based on palm kernel oil and hydrogenated soybean and cottonseed oils. The *Freedom* line is an ideal alternative to hydrogenated coatings used in bakery and the healthy snack bar industries. All are *trans*-free and offer a lower saturated fat content than the standard palm kernel type coatings. They are designed to be bloom-free for the shelf life of most baked goods, and are compatible with current bakery shortenings and palm based shortenings.

For food products that are promoted as "healthy," Loders Croklaan provides no-*trans* solutions that have a reduced saturated fat content. *Sanstrans* HF has the same functionality as *Sanstrans* 39 or 42, with 15% less saturated fat. For maximum saturated fat reduction use the Loders Croklaan hardstock approach. Hardstock fats are blended with non-hydrogenated liquid oils at low levels, and entrap large amounts of liquid oil resulting in a shortenings with about 30% saturates. The standard hardstock for baking is *Sanstrans* LS, and a less waxy version for premium applications called *Sanstrans* MG.

TABLE 4

Freedom Coating Fats

Product	Melting point °C/F	Type	Typical applications
Freedom 340	43/109	Flexible coating fat	For use in all coated bakery products, including cookies, donuts, cakes and donuts
Freedom 540	43/109	Hard coating fat	Firm coating fat for baked goods and snack bars
Freedom 875	41/106	Flexible coating fat	Rapid crystallizing coating fat for baked goods and bars
Freedom 900 series	—	Hard coating fat	A range of palm kernel based coating fats suitable for snack bars and confections

Loders Croklaan provides comprehensive technical service and custom product manufacture for difficult applications. For further information about our compete range of no-*trans* solutions, visit our web-site at www.Sans*trans*.com.

Gerald P. McNeill
Loders Croklaan
24708 West Durkee Road
Channahon, IL 60410
gerald.mcneill@croklaan.com

Premium Vegetable Oils Sdn Bhd

Novel Non-Hydrogenated Hard Palm Fraction and *Trans*-Free Structural Fat

Traditionally, hard stocks for the manufacture of oils and fats products that require solid consistency such as margarine, spread or shortening are made using hydrogenated oils or a blend of hydrogenated oils with liquid oils. Even fat blends suitable for the production of liquid frying oils and fluid shortening are hydrogenated to increase their stability by removing or reducing 18:3 fatty acids. Although increased product stability may be obtained by partial hydrogenation, this process introduces man-made *trans* fatty acids (TFA).

It is theoretically true that if oils and fats are fully hydrogenated then zero TFA levels can be achieved. However, consumers often simply equate hydrogenation with TFA. Hence many manufacturers are looking for a "clean" label on their ingredient list that does not include hydrogenated fats.

Palm oil and its fractions can be used alone or as blends with liquid oils to produce products with higher solid fat profiles. This reduces the level of TFA in the products to practically negligible levels. However, incorporation of palm fractions results in an increased saturated fatty acid (SAFA) level in the products, depending upon the percentage incorporation of palm oil fractions and the hydrogenated oil replaced.

Following nutritional guidance from government nutritionists, consumers now look for products not only with low TFA levels but also with low SAFA levels. Food companies, in turn, look for non-hydrogenated, low-SAFA fat systems having a low 18:3 level to ensure high oxidative stability.

Research has therefore been carried out to develop healthier hardstock alternatives that contain no hydrogenated oils while at the same time providing functional performance equal to or better than the hydrogenated hard stocks which they replace. The healthier final product is achieved by simultaneously reducing the SAFA level in the total fat blend. By judicious choice of non hydrogenated hard lauric oil and palm oil fractions followed by interesterification, the resultant fat produced will have optimum levels of H_3 as well as H_2M type triglycerides present in them ("H" denotes a saturated fatty acid residue having carbon chain length of 16 and above and "M" for 14 and below). Hardstocks of this type may then be blended at low levels with various liquid oils to produce blends with low SAFA fat levels but good product functionality.

Premium's patented (U.S. 6,808,737), novel, non-hydrogenated *trans*-free hard structural fat products—Magfat series—have been found to have excellent structuring effects even at very low level usage with liquid oils (Table 1). Using such *trans*-free hardstocks, manufacturers are in a position to achieve not only extremely low

TABLE 1
Main characteristics of Premium's Magfat products

Test	Magfat 30	Magfat 50	Magfat CAF 50
SMP°C	51.0	45.8	46.8
SFC @			
20°C	86.1	95.3	96.3
25°C	78.6	86.2	91.8
30°C	66.5	74.2	83.8
35°C	52.1	55.9	69.7
40°C	34.7	34.4	48.6
%-SAFA	88.5	91.8	92.9
%-MUFA	9.7	6.9	5.9
%-PUFA	1.8	1.3	1.2

trans levels, but also low SAFA levels—all without having to label the product as containing hydrogenated oil. In short, by using these novel fats, food companies can achieve "clean and green" product labels that attract today's demanding consumers.

To illustrate what may be achieved with Premium's patented Magfat, we have benchmarked Becel™ margarine for the purpose of comparison. The average test results of samples collected from the market are given in the tables below.

Table 2 shows results for Magfat CAF 50 blended with soybean oil. An addition of between 5 and 10% Magfat CAF 50 is sufficient to provide the same SFC profile as in Becel™ with similar SAFA. Tables 3 and 4 shows blends with canola oil as well as high-oleic canola oil which results in even lower SAFA. By choice of the liquid oil—soy, canola, sun, etc.—the balance of mono-unsaturated fatty acids (MUFA) and and polyunsaturated fatty acids (PUFA) may be adjusted as required.

Table 4 shows the use of Magfat 50. This hardstock is less functional than Magfat CAF 50 meaning that a little more is required for the same SFCs. Nevertheless it can be seen that at the 10% addition level a product very similar to Becel™ can be obtained.

If no lauric oils are desired, then Premium's patented (US 6,808,737), hard palm stearin fraction, Margo, having a palmitic acid level of 75–87% may be interesterified with liquid vegetable oils to produce designer fats with low SAFA as well as

TABLE 2
Blend Study: Magfat CAF 50 and Soybean Oil (SBO)

Blend (%)		SMP	Solid Fat Content (%)						Fatty Acids (%)		
SBO	Magfat CAF 50	°C	10°C	20°C	25°C	30°C	35°C	40°C	SAFA	MUFA	PUFA
100	0	3.0	—	—	—	—	—	—			
95	5	28.0	6.0	3.2	2.1	1.4	0.6	—	18.4	21.7	59.9
90	10	33.6	11.7	7.3	5.4	3.8	2.2	0.2	22.3	21	57
85	15	35.2	16.9	11.5	8.6	6.3	3.8	1.5	26.1	20	50.9
Becel™		31.2	6.8	4.7	3.3	2.4	1.6	—	14.9	47.0	38.1

TABLE 3
Blend Study: Magfat CAF 50 and Canola Oil

Blend (%)		SMP	Solid Fat Content (%)						Fatty Acids (%)		
Canola	Magfat CAF 50	°C	10°C	20°C	25°C	30°C	35°C	40°C	SAFA	MUFA	PUFA
—	100.0	48.0	96.8	95.9	91.8	82.6	68.3	47.9	92.9	5.9	1.2
80.0	20.0	33.2	18.6	13.6	11.1	8.5	5.5	3.0	23.9	53.4	22.7
85.0	15.0	27.6	13.2	9.6	7.6	5.6	3.5	1.6	19.6	56.4	24.1
90.0	10.0	22.8	8.3	6.0	4.5	3.3	1.7	0.3	15.2	59.4	25.4
95.0	5.0	10.4	3.7	2.4	1.7	1.0	0.1	nil	10.9	62.3	26.8
100.0	—	—	—	—	—	—	—	—	6.6	65.3	28.1
Becel™		31.2	6.8	4.7	3.3	2.4	1.6	—	14.9	47.0	38.1

TABLE 4
Blend Study: Magfat CAF 50 and High—Oleic Canola Oil (HCO)

Blend (%)		SMP	Solid Fat Content (%)						Fatty Acids (%)		
HCO	Magfat CAF 50	°C	10°C	20°C	25°C	30°C	35°C	40°C	SAFA	MUFA	PUFA
100	0	—	—	—	—	—	—	—	6.1	77.9	16
95	5	10.4	3.7	2.4	1.7	1.0	0.1	—	10.4	74.4	15.2
90	10	22.8	8.3	5.9	4.6	3.3	1.7	0.3	14.7	70.8	14.5
85	15	27.6	13.2	9.6	7.6	5.6	3.5	1.6	19.1	67.2	13.7
Becel™		31.2	6.8	4.7	3.3	2.4	1.6	—	14.9	47.0	38.1

enough solid levels to produce edible plastic products. In Table 5 are shown blends which would be suitable for industrial margarines or shortenings. By choice of the liquid oil—high oleic sun, canola, rice bran oil, etc., the 18:3 levels may be adjusted as required

By blending Magfat at slightly increased levels with selected liquid oils, shortening with low SAFA levels can be produced. Blend studies with sunflower oil, high oleic sunflower oil, rice bran oil, etc., have been carried out and has been found that

TABLE 5
Blend Study: Magfat 50 and High-Oleic Canola Oil (HCO)

Blend (%)		SMP	Solid Fat Content (%)						Fatty Acids (%)		
HCO	Magfat 50	°C	10°C	20°C	25°C	30°C	35°C	40°C	SAFA	MUFA	PUFA
100	0	—	—	—	—	—	—	—	6.1	77.9	16
95	5	14.0	3.5	2.1	1.4	0.6	—	—	10.4	74.4	15.2
90	10	24.0	7.7	5.0	3.6	2.3	1.4	—	14.5	71.0	14.5
85	15	28.0	12.3	8.2	6.5	4.6	2.8	0.8	18.7	67.5	13.8
BecelTM		31.2	6.8	4.7	3.3	2.4	1.6	—	14.9	47.0	38.1

TABLE 6
Blend / Interesterification Study—Margo with Soybean Oil (SBO)

Test	Margo	SBO	Margo:SBO (20:80)		Margo:SBO (10:90)	
			Before IE	After IE	Before IE	After IE
IV	13.2	130.0	103.1	103.6	114.7	115.0
SMP °C	60.0	3.0	49.4	48.4	44.6	42.0
SFC @						
10°C	94.6	0.2	22.4	21.1	11.7	10.7
20°C	93.7	—	18.3	16.8	8.9	7.5
25°C	91.7		15.9	14.6	7.6	5.9
30°C	88.1		13.7	12.5	6.4	4.8
35°C	83.3		11.7	10.5	4.9	3.7
40°C	75.6		9.3	8.2	3.4	2.4

For further enquiries please contact pvoamericas@qtm.net or visit our website www.premiumveg.com.

the Magfat series hard stocks are excellent to produce margarine, spreads, shortening, etc., with low SAFA levels.

U.R. Sahasranamam
Premium Vegetable Oils Sdn Bhd
27th Floor, Wisma Tun Sanbandan
Jalan SultanSulaiman
50000, Kuala Lumpur
Malaysia
urs@premium-kl.com

Index

A

Aarhus United USA, 107–109
  Cisao, 108
  Cebes® NH, 108–109
  EsSense, 107–108
Activist groups, 98
  BanTransFat.com, 98
  Center for Science in the Public Interest, 98
ADM NovaLipids, 110–113
  blending, 111
  enzymatic interesterification, 112–113
  lauric and palm fats, 110–111
  naturally stable oils, 110
Alternatives to hydrogenation, 73–74
American Heart Association, 98
ANPR, *see Trans* Fat Advance Notice of Proposed Rulemaking
Applications, 83–84
Asymmetric di-acid TAG, 21
  molecular packing and properties of, 21
ATR-FTIR Official Method AOCS Cd 14d-99/AOAC 2000.10, 63–65

B

"Bad" cholesterol (LDL), 34
Blood cholesterol levels, 26
Bunge Oils, 114–116
  NH line of products, 115
    Anhydrous NH Roll–In Shortening, 115
    Bakers Ideal® NH Pastry Margarine, 115
    Coral® NH Margarine, 115
    Cremol® NH Specialty Icing Shortening, 115
    Croissant NH Margarine, 115
    NH Biscuit Flakes, 115
    Summit® 40 NH Pastry Margarine, 115
    Super Cel® NH Specialty Cake Shortening, 115
    Tri-Co®NH Emulsified Dough Shortening, 115
    Victor® NH Bakers Grade Margarine, 115
    Vream® NH All Purpose Shortening, 115
    Vreamay® NH Cake & Icing Shortening, 115
  RighT™ line of products, 114–115
    Victor *RighT*™ Margarine, 114
    Vream *RighT*™ All Purpose Shortening, 114
    Vreamay *RighT*™ Cake and Icing Shortening, 114
  Specialty oils, 115–116
    Nutra Clear HS™ Canola Oil, 115–116
    NUTRIUM™ Low Linolenic Soybean Oil, 116

C

Cargill, in *trans* fat regulations, 117–118
  Zero *trans* Liquid Oils, 117
  Zero *trans* Solid Shortenings, 118
Challenges, 72
Chemical structures for common fatty acids, 48
  in fats and oils, 47
CHD, *see* Coronary heart disease
Cis configuration, 2, 4
Clinical trials involving TFA, 38–41
Cocoa butter, 6
  melting behavior, 7
Commercial solutions, 106–127
Consumer knowledge, 99–102
Consumer perceptions, 98
Consumer questions about *trans* fat, 92–95
Consumer response to breakfast cereal survey, 102
Coronary heart disease, 26

D

Daily Reference Value, 26
Designer fats, 15–17
    molecular packing and polymorphism,
        15–17
Determination of *trans* fats by gas
    chromatography and infrared
    methods, 47–68
Dietary guidelines, processing
    and reformulation for *trans*
    reduction, 71–84
Dietary Guidelines 2000, 28
Dietary guidelines for Americans 2005,
    71–72
Dietary level of TFA, 38–44
    clinical trials, 36–44
Dietary recommendations, 34, 41–44
    saturated fatty acids, 34
    trans fatty acids, 34
Dietary recommendations: non–U.S.
    organizations, 43
    Austria, Germany, Switzerland,
        43, 44
    Health Canada, 43
    Health Council of The Netherlands, 43
    Ministry of Agriculture, UK,
        43, 44
    World Health Organization/Food
        and Agricultural Organization
        of the United Nations, 43, 44
Dietary recommendations: U.S.
    organizations, 42
    American Heart Association, 42
    National Cholesterol Education
        Program, 42
    Institute of Medicine/National Academy
        of Sciences, 42
Dietary Reference Intake, 26
Dietary *trans* fatty acids, 34
    blood lipid parameters, 34
DRI, *see* Dietary Reference Intake
DRV, *see* Daily Reference Value
Dry fractionation, 78–79
    olein, 78
    palm oil, 78
    stearine, 78

E

Energy, 39
    as TFA, 39
    as linoleic acid in TFA diet treatments, 39
Enzymatic interesterification, 75–77

F

Fats, 5
    oxidative stability, 5
    physical properties, 15
    solid fat functionality, 5
Fatty acid composition, 3, 13
    of conventional oils, 3
    of high oleic oils, 3
    of palm oil, palm fractions, 13
Fatty acids, 2
    monounsaturated, 2
    polyunsaturated, 2
Fatty acid structures, 1–2
FDA regulations, 23,
Fluid shortenings, 80
Food and Drug Administration Labeling
    Rule, 25
Food label declaration, 30
Food company responses, 99
Food product label, 12
    trans fat content in ingredient, 12
    fat/serving, 12
Formulation, 9–10
    addition of antioxidants to fats
        and oils, 9
    blending partially hydrogenated fat, 9
    entrapment of liquid oils, 9
    modified (special) hydrogenation
        conditions, 10
    use of palm fractions, 9
Fourier-transform infrared spectroscopy,
    55–57
    instrumentation, 55–57
Fractionation, 12–13
    solvent, 12
    dry, 12
FTIR, *see* Fourier-transform infrared
    spectroscopy
FTIR instrumentation, 57

Functional fat, 15
  nutrition/health characteristics, 15
Functional need for solid fat, 4
  in food products, 4
  instead of oils, 5
  nutrition/health characteristics, 15
Functional properties of oils and fats, 5
  hardness, 5
  mouth feel, 5
  oxidative stability, 5

G

Genetics, 10
Glycerol backbone, 1
Glycerol conformation, 21–23
  in molecular packing and properties, 21–23
"Good" cholesterol (HDL), 34

H

HDL-cholesterol, "good" cholesterol, 34
High stability oils, 80–81
How to reformulate, 102–104
How not to reformulate, 104–105
HSO, *see* high stability oils
Hydrogenation, 10
  conditions, 11
  processes, 11

I

Interesterification, 13–15
  chemical, 14
Institute of Medicine, 26, 27
IOM, *see* Institute of Medicine
IOM/NAS report, 27–28
Isomerism, 4
  cis, 4
  trans, 4

L

Labeling of TFA in foods, 47
LDL-cholesterol, "bad" cholesterol, 34, 41
  levels based on diet, 38

change in LDL-Cholesterol with level
    of dietary TFA, 41
LDL/HDL ratio, 38–41
  change with level of dietary linoleic
    acid, 40
Loders Croklaan, 119–123
  palm oil alternative to *trans* fat, 119–123
  supply and cost, 119
  palm oil functionality, 119
  palm oil products
    Freedom coating fats, 120, 122–123
    Sanstrans oils and shortenings,
      120–122

M

Margarine, relative distribution of *trans*
    C18:1 positional isomers, 49
Medical costs, 98
Melting temperatures and enthalpies, 18, 20
  of di-acid symmetrical TAG, 20, 22
  of asymmetric TAG, 22
  of single acid TAG, 18
  of OSO
  of OOS
Molecular structures, 8
  elaidic acid, 8
  oleic acid, 8
  stearic acid, 8
Monoacid TAG, 17
  molecular packing and properties
    of, 17–18

N

National Academy of Sciences (NAS),
    26, 27
National Cholesterol Education Program, 28
National Association of Margarine
    Manufacturers, 35
NCEP, *see* National Cholesterol Education
    Program
No *trans* fats, 73
  coconut, 73
  corn, 73
  cottonseed, 73
  high oleic canola, 73

high oleic safflower, 73
high oleic sunflower, 73
low linolenic soybean oils, 73
mid oleic sunflower, 73
palm, 73
palm kernel, 73
Nutritional considerations
    of *trans* fatty acids, 34–44
Nutrient content and health
        claims, 27
Nutrition facts labels, 89, 91
Nutrition Facts panel, 26
    changes to, 26
Nutrition labeling, 26
Nutrition Labeling and Education Act
        of 1990, 26, 71

O

Official methods, 51–68
    Capillary gas chromatography,
        51–52
    GC Official Methods AOAC 996.06,
        52–53
    AOCS Ce 1f-96, 52–53
    status and limitations of, 65–68
Oils, 2–6
    coconut, 2
    palm, 2
    palm kernel, 2
    soybean, 3, 7
    tropical, 2
Oils with modified composition, 79–80
Oxidation, 5
    rates, 5

P

Palm oil fractionation, 13
Partial GC FAME profile in AOCS
        Ce 1f-96, 59
Partial hydrogenation, 73
Patent literature, 75–76
Phase behavior, 19
    of EEE, 19
    of SSS, 19
    of di-acid triacylglycerol, 20

Prefractionation of *trans* C18:1 geometric
        isomers by silver ion
        chromatography, 54–55
Premium Vegetable Oils Sdn Bhd, 124–127
    novel non-hydrogenated hard palm
        fraction and *trans*-free structural
        fat, 124–127
Properties and sources of *trans,* 7

Q

Quantitative GC determination of *trans* fatty
        acids, 53–54

R

Ranges of *trans* fat contents in selected food
        products, 49RBD oils, 1
Recent human dietary studies involving
        TFA re: blood lipoproteins, 36–41
Reformulation, 74–81
    blending hard/soft feed stocks, 74–75
    chemical/enzymatic interesterification,
        74–75
    fractionation, 74–75
    genetic/plant breeding, 74–75
    modified hydrogenation, 74–75
Reformulation for reduced TFA
        content, 82
Relative distribution of *trans* C18:1
        positional isomers, 50
    in cow milk, 50
    in human milk, 50
Reproducibility relative standard deviation,
        RSD(R), 66

S

Saturated fatty acids, 2
    lauric, 2
    myristic, 2
    palmitic, 2
    stearic, 2
SFC, *see* solid fat content
SFI, *see* solid fat index
Shortening oils, 75
sn-glycerol derivatives, 1

Solid fat content, 6
Solid fat index, 6
Spreads containing a *trans* fat footnote, 90
Structure and occurrence of *trans* fatty
    acids, 47–50
Successful communication, 90–92
    points to consider, 90–92
Symmetric di-acid TAG, 18
    molecular packing and properties of,
        18–21

T

TAG, *see* triacylglycerols
TFA in U.S. Food Supply, 34
    occurrence, 34–36
Trans configuration, 2, 4
Trans Fat Advance Notice of Proposed
    Rulemaking, 30–31
Trans Fat Final Rule, 28–30
Trans fat labeling proposed rule, 26–28
Trans fat
    content per serving size, 12
    importance of consumer research, 87–95
    new FDA regulations, 26–31
Trans fat footnote on nutrition facts label,
    87–90
    consumer weighting of information,
        88–90
Trans fat infrared methodology, 60–62
Trans fats, 1–25,
    chemistry, 1
    intakes, re: coronary heart disease, 28
    intakes, re: dietary patterns, 28
    occurrence, 1
    overview, 1–4
    properties, 7
    reduction technologies, 9
    regulations, 9
    sources, 7, 8
Trans fat reduction in foods/oils, 72
Trans fat reformulation, 96–105
Trans fats reduction/elimination
    technologies, 9
Trans fatty acids (TFA), 34, 35
    in blood lipoproteins, 36–38
    in food fats, 35

    in products, 35
    typical levels, 35
"*Trans* free" status, 96
Trans reduction by modified hydrogenation,
    81–82
Trans TFA and saturated acid content
    of hydrogenated soy oil based food
    oils, 83
Transesterification, 14
Transmission FTIR Official Method AOCS
    Cd 14-95/AOAC 965.34, 62–63
Transmission mode, 57–60
    Attenuated total reflection mode,
        58–60
Typical levels of trans fatty acids in food
    fats/products, 35
    beef and dairy fat, 35
    frying fats, 35
    margarines/spreads, 35
    shortenings, 35

U

Unsaturated fatty acids, 2
    linoleic, 2
    linolenic, 2
    oleic, 2

V

Vegetable oils, 8
    partial hydrogenation, 8
Vegetable oils of commerce, 1
    soybean, 1
    cottonseed, 1
    canola, 1
    sunflower, 1
    corn, 1
    peanut, 1
    palm, 1
    palm kernel, 1
    coconut, 1

Z

Zero *trans* margarines/shortenings, 75